HE DID IT!

"If you learned to be fat, you can learn to be thin."
Dr. Laurence Reich knows what he is talking about
when he shows overweight men and women how to
change themselves from fat to skinny—for good.
He did it himself. By following the simple, enjoyable
program contained in this book, he changed himself
from a 300-pound "eating loser" to a 162-pound
"eating winner."

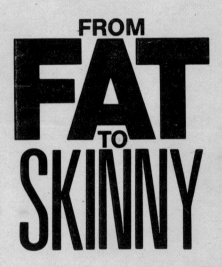

FROM
FAT
TO
SKINNY

"How he accomplished this miracle through his
eating habits and thought patterns is told with
such cheerful aplomb that the overweight reader
is compelled to action. . . . fascinating reading."

LOS ANGELES TIMES

FROM
FAT
TO
SKINNY

DR. LAURENCE REICH

PLAYBOY PRESS
PAPERBACKS

Names and identifying details
have been changed throughout this book
to assure the privacy of those concerned.

Published simultaneously in the United States and Canada by Playboy Press, Chicago, Illinois. Printed in the United States of America. Wyden Books hardcover edition published 1977. Playboy Press soft-cover edition published 1979.

Books are available at quantity discounts for promotional and indus-rial use. For further information, write our sales promotion agency: Ventura Associates, 40 East 49th Street, New York, New York 10017.

ISBN: 0-872-16509-4

Contents

Acknowledgments

To all those people and places who supported my change and assisted me in its description.

To Marian and Gus: for their dedication to the parenting process—it's working.

To Gail, Jeff, Dana, and Tracy: for their bottomless chocolate-chip cookie closet—I don't need it any more.

To Davita and Stu: for all the love, support, and sharing—it just goes on.

To Abe Maslow: for movement toward the attainment of the best there is.

To Michelle: for nurturing support and guidance throughout the entire change process.

To Sultan: for ultimate courage and a lesson in terror and aliveness—once was enough.

To Werner: for clarity on boredom—it only gives you something to do.

To Jeanne and Jerry: for the sharing of our lives—it just continues to grow.

To Barry: for controlled patience beyond sartorial guidance.

To the New York cuisinaholics: Abe, Jean, and Duncan, for the never-ending feasts.

To Piero Dimitri, sartorial couturier without exception: for allowing me into your factory and the fulfillment of yet another possible dream.

To Verne: for corporate courage to support the unusual and the unique.

To Donna P. and Laurie A.: for courage to experience the change process from a different point of view.

To Tina, Jason, and Les: for the love and support while growing thin.

To Pat, Bill, and Peter: for from there to here—noticing what could be.

To Wilkes Bashford, individually and collectively: for the experience—distinctive, unique, and expansive.

To the Dimitri showroom and factory staff, and of course his models, hairdressers, and photographers: for the experience of being with you—"the gynecologist."

To Diane and Tom Kron: for the best chocolate nipples—I'm pacified.

To Richard Simmons: for salads with style—what a service.

To Linda Lewis: for the raspberry swirls—they sustain the pictures.

To Maurice Bonté: for all that is succulent.

To Raina: for the innocence of youth and the creativity it supports.

And to great green cucumbers and long cool zucchini: for whatever your rewards may be.

To the process of change; and to those who are willing to be courageous and creative so as to facilitate its purposeful occurrence.

And

For Ron Pion who transcended the shadow long ago—you stand alone.

FROM FAT TO SKINNY

1

A Set of Contrasts

The time is about two and a half years ago. The place is New York City. The setting is a well-known, very fashionable French restaurant. It is just after eight-thirty in the evening. Four men are seated at one of the tables. They happen to be obstetrician-gynecologists who live and practice in Honolulu. For the past ten days they have been attending a conference dealing with new therapeutic techniques in sex and reproduction. This is their last evening in New York. In the morning, they fly back to Honolulu. Dinner at this particular restaurant is their way of winding up a valuable and informative conference. It is a sort of going away/going home present—a nice treat. There is nothing out of the ordinary about the four men, but one of them is taller and noticeably heavier than his companions. In fact, he is plain fat—three hundred pounds fat.

All four men are almost finished with the main course. They treated themselves well and covered all courses, especially the fat diner. He started out with an order of onion soup dripping with melted cheese. Then he ate a fresh spinach salad tossed with crumbled bacon and croutons and topped with a rich, creamy dressing. Four varieties of bread were placed on the table. The fat fellow tried all four. His entrée of chicken in wine sauce has been consumed. There is nothing left to eat on his plate, but bits and pieces are left on the other plates.

The four doctors are not talking shop. Rather, they are chatting about the plans they have for the weekend. One is talking about the Japanese garden he and his wife are building and the trouble they are having with the installation of the fish pond. The fat fellow is not really paying attention to the conversation. His attention is drawn to a piece of uneaten châteaubriand lying in a pool of béarnaise sauce. At this moment, he couldn't care less about fish ponds; he wants that piece of meat his colleague shows no sign of eating. How to get at it is his prime concern, but he just cannot bring himself to spear the meat with his fork in full view of his companions.

Suddenly, one of the doctors interrupts the fish pond story to announce, "Will you look at who's walking in!" Four pairs of eyes turn toward the door. One of the world's most famous women and her party are being escorted to the best table in the dining room. Since doctors are just as celebrity conscious as the next person, all, except the fat guy, watch closely.

The celebrity distraction has given him the chance he needs. Quick as a flash, he spears the meat with his fork. A part of the châteaubriand is in his mouth and down his throat, with the next piece on its way, before the other three turn their attention back to the table and each other. No one seems to notice the "châteaubriand snatch."

Wheeling a tray of French pastries, a solicitous waiter suggests dessert. Only two of the diners agree, the fatty and one other doctor. The overweight doctor selects a thick slice of cheese cake topped with fresh raspberry sauce, and his companion decides on a *crème marron* laced with sherry. All four ask for coffee and brandy. With all the ceremony for which the restaurant is known, the food and drink are placed on the table. The fat doctor digs right in, but his companion in dessert abandons the goodie after a few nibbles. "What's the matter with the *crème marron*?" the fat guy asks.

"Nothing. It's too sweet for my taste, that's all," he explains.

"Well, you can't let it go to waste. You're going to pay for it anyway. I'll eat it for you," the overweight doctor volunteers.

"Fine. Go ahead."

So a second dessert is polished off, and both are washed down with coffee with two sugars and a generous lacing of heavy cream. About twenty minutes later the four men settle their bill and stroll back to their hotel. Once in the lobby, they decide to wind up the evening. One wants to finish packing, and two others want to get to bed early. The fourth one, our heavy friend, does not have any particular plans and mumbles something about buying a few magazines to read on the plane.

Actually, the fatty does not know what to do with himself. His packing is done, there is nothing very interesting on television, and it is too early for bed. After seeing his colleagues safely into the elevator, he turns and strolls with exaggerated casualness into the hotel's all-night coffee shop, where he does buy two magazines. One of the cover stories seems interesting. He wants to read it right away, and since the chair in his room is not very comfortable, he decides to stay where he is. Gazing around the coffee shop, he notices comfortable-looking booths toward the rear wall. He settles into one and opens the magazine.

A waitress comes over and sets the table; pleasantly, efficiently, she flips open her order pad. What can the poor guy do? Coffee shops are for eating, not reading. So he orders a piece of banana cream pie and a vanilla malted. Deeply engrossed in the article, he hardly notices what he is eating, but he eats.

After he finishes the article, he pays his bill at the cashier's; he also picks up two chocolate-covered peanut rolls and a roll of assorted fruit-flavored lifesavers from the display rack alongside the cash register. Back in his room, he switches on the eleven o'clock news and munches on the candy bars as he watches. When the news is over, the tubby takes a quick shower and gets into bed. The bed groans a bit as he settles his three hundred pounds into a comfortable position, but that does not bother him; he has heard those sounds before. Soon he drifts off to sleep.

The next morning he is up bright and early, bright and early enough so he is dressed and downstairs before his friends. Rather than wait around in the lobby, he heads for the coffee shop again. The rules have not changed. He cannot say to the waitress, "I'm just waiting for my friends," so he orders a breakfast of orange juice, a cheese and mushroom omelet, bacon, toast with butter and blackberry jelly, and coffee with milk and sugar. While he eats, he scans the morning paper. When his three companions drift in, this fellow is just wiping up the last traces of melted cheese with a bit of toast. Because they are taking a breakfast flight, the other doctors order only juice and coffee.

About two hours later, the foursome is in a plane to Honolulu. A stewardess is serving breakfast—warmish juice, sausage patties, soggy pancakes with syrup, and coffee with milk and sugar. All four dig in. Three are really having their breakfast, but the fat one is on his second feeding. Even though the food is typical mediocre airline fare, he devours every morsel, including the sweet puddle of excess syrup.

This scenario could be continued, but I do not think it is necessary. You have a picture of a man, a fat man, who makes a hog of himself with food. Given the opportunity, he is a nonstop fork-lift-to-mouth man.

The scene now shifts to another restaurant, this time in Honolulu. About eighteen months have passed. Three couples are gathered for dinner and have now finished. At first glance there is nothing unusual about the six men and women at the table, but a closer look shows one man, a tall man who weighs about 162 pounds, still eating—even though his dinner was only a salad: a very appetizing salad—a pale orange papaya surrounded by a banana, a mango, and a creamy white d'anjou pear resting on a bed of cool, crisp Manoa lettuce and topped with rich yogurt dressing. The others at the table are waiting for him, but not impatiently, to finish. Each time he lifts his fork to his mouth, he chews slowly and deliberately, savoring the different flavors of the fruits. Between bites he puts his fork down and joins in the conversation. He is enjoying himself—the company, the food, the conversation.

Finally he finishes, and a waiter approaches to clear the table and take the dessert order. Everybody but the man who had the salad orders something. He passes up dessert because he is full—he is not going to eat for the sake of eating; black coffee will be enough to complete his meal. Over dessert and coffee the gay chatter continues. One of the women pushes a half-eaten dish of ice cream to one side. The man who passed up dessert notices and does nothing about it.

Like the previous scenario, this one could be expanded, but there is no need to do so. You have a picture of a man who is in control of his eating pattern. He can enjoy and feel satisfied with a light meal; he can say no to food he is not truly hungry for and still have a grand time. He pays more attention to the life around him than to the food.

Are you saying, "It must be wonderful to be like that"? Speaking from personal experience, I can answer that it most certainly is—because the two men, the one stuffing himself in New York and the one just described, have the same name: Larry Reich.

Yes, there was a time when I weighed about three hundred pounds. That was the old me—the fat me operating on automatic pilot. The new thin me operates primarily on manual pilot. This was one of the ways I achieved a quick weight loss.

How did I make the switch? How can you make the switch? It is not hard, and it does not involve pills, obesity specialists, or diet groups. Just learning something new so you can change your eating pattern from automatic to manual and from fat to thin. It is not difficult at all. It is a bit awkward at first, but learning a new activity always involves an initial period of awkwardness. Actually, there is an excellent chance you will find losing weight to be fun, because learning has tremendous enjoyment potential. Certainly losing weight is an adventure. Learning is something anybody, and I mean anybody, can do. It does not take a special talent of any sort. After all, if you learned to be fat, and you and I did learn to be fat, you can learn to be thin.

2

What This Book Is All About

This book is essentially about learning—with a specific emphasis on learning to be thin. I want the book to assist you in learning so by extension you can learn how to be thin. Losing weight and keeping it off involves learning. Before you close this book with an "Okay, that's it. This guy is not for me. I'm too busy for all this jazz," hear me out.

I do not know how many people have cut me off in mid-sentence to say, "Me? Learn? I'm too dumb," or "too old," or "learning is too hard." Anything but this is the case. Every-body, anybody—you, me, ordinary people—is capable of acquiring new knowledge, new behavior, and new points of view. And this is what learning is all about.

A lot of people are also turned off by the subject of learn-ing because they associate learning with school. A lot of people do not like school. The thought of a classroom situa-tion brings up visions of having to sit quietly at a desk and listen. Well, this ain't school.

Yet I can understand and sympathize with your doubts about learning how to change a point of view. There was a time when I, too, believed a point of view could not be changed. When I was in medical school I learned a great deal about the diagnosis and treatment of disease. To my mind, medicine concentrated on the negative—sickness. Health did not excite interest, disease did. I was not happy with this point of view, but I did not realize I could change it.

Then I met a doctor, Ron Pion, whose attitude was the exact opposite. Ron is an obstetrician-gynecologist whose specialty was working with people who had sexual and/or reproductive problems. While this field was interesting and exciting to me, even more so was Ron's point of view. He was not content merely to treat sickness or disease, but rather, stressed a positive outlook as the path to good health.

Because of my association with Ron Pion, I learned how to change my point of view. Today I see medicine can be a positive force—not only preventing illness and curing it but promoting health and well-being as well. This is just one example of something that changed my way of thinking. Now let's talk about you and *your* vast, possibly untapped, ability to learn. Because whether you realize it or not, you can learn.

I believe, with few exceptions, that everyone is capable of growing, expanding, changing—in other words, of learning. The best proof of your learning abilities is the very fact you are reading this book. Were you born able to read or were you taught as a child? Could you always tie your shoes, drive a car, run a washing machine, operate a power tool, use a typewriter? The answer has to be no. But you learned to do things like this. Think for a moment. Can you do something today you could not do two months ago? If you can learn to do one thing, you can also learn to do other things—like being thin.

Usually most people do not give themselves credit for being able to learn because once a skill has been learned, it is taken for granted. I guess all of us know how to tie our shoes, and I also suspect most people take this skill for granted. Imagine for a moment, though, that your hands are crippled with arthritis. Would you then find tying shoes so easy?

Along with learning, this book also deals with change: why

many of us find change scary, why we build barriers to prevent change—but more important, how we *can* change, and what benefits we can derive from change.

"What if I don't want to change, then what?" you may be asking. I might respond, "In what way don't you want to change?"

There is change, and there is change. Whatever the change, we are usually unprepared for it. We cannot foresee the outcome, and so most of us find it threatening. That is, until after the change has been accomplished. Before and during the process, we tend to see change from a negative point of view. Once the change has been accomplished, we tend to alter that view—generally toward the positive.

Moving is a good example. Most people are not pleased when they have to move. The packing. The confusion. New schools for the kids. New neighbors to meet. The point of view is negative. But let six months go by . . . Everything is unpacked and order is restored. The kids make new friends. The neighbors turn out to be swell. Suddenly the change does not seem so negative. In fact, the evaluation generally becomes positive. Change has been accomplished.

Yet we live with change all our lives. We have all changed physically and will continue to do so. We have gone from infants to children to adolescents to adults. You have probably gone from thin to fat and maybe from fat to fatter. This is change in the physical sense. We have also changed emotionally. Does your teddy bear mean the same to you today as it did when you were a child? Does the idol of your teenage years still interest you? Do you like doing today the same things you loved ten or twenty years ago? Do you enjoy something today that just a few short years ago you thought you would always dislike? All these are emotional changes.

Let me ask my question again: "In what way don't you want to change?" Your spouse, your job, your politics, your religion, your hair color? If this is what you mean, put your doubts to rest. I have no intention of browbeating you to change anything. But what about your weight? Do *you want* to change your weight?

"That's a ridiculous question!" you are probably thinking to yourself. "Of course I want to lose weight. I'm reading this book." Yes, you are reading this book, and that pleases me. I wrote this book so people would read it. But my question, and it is not so ridiculous, still stands. Do you really want to lose weight?

And more important—who wants you to lose weight? Do *you*? Or is someone else hassling you? Your spouse, your kids, your employer? If *you* want to lose weight, slimming down is easy. But if someone else is on your back, losing can be tough! Being fat is not so bad if you are satisfied with your weight. And if you are pleased with your weight, that is all that matters.

To answer my questions, consider asking yourself what you think you might gain by being thinner. There are some advantages that thin people have that I know about. Thin people never have trouble buckling seatbelts, and they never have to squeeze into seats at the movies or on an airplane. Thin people can sit on a fragile antique chair without having the owner turning white and thinking, "If you break that chair, I'll break you." Thin people can buy clothes that fit them—they do not have to settle for anything that covers them.

These advantages apply only to some people. Maybe you do not care about clothes. Even if you weighed one hundred pounds less, you would still wear blue jeans and T-shirts. Maybe you never go to the movies, so the width of the seats does not interest you. Seat belts, antique furniture, and getting in and out of compact cars may not play any part in your life.

So what do *you* expect to gain from your weight loss? A longer life? Better health? Statistics do seem to bear out the fact that thinner people have fewer problems with such vital organs as the heart and the lungs; and supposedly, the thinner you are, the healthier you are.

I cannot promise that if you lose weight you will live longer. Maybe you will; but even if you do, other factors may be the cause of your longevity, and not your weight loss. Many people come from families with a history of longevity. Some people believe that genes have a lot to do with how long you live. Maybe, too, the day you achieve your weight goal you could be hit by a truck. I cannot (nobody can) promise a longer, healthier life because of a loss in weight. It would seem, however, that fat or thin, even if you live to be one hundred and one, your life will be too short to suit you. Most people, when they go, are not ready for it.

Do you think that if you lose weight, you will be happier? Possibly you will be, but perhaps you are happy now. I have met fat people who are genuinely happy with their lives and their weight. I have also met thin people who were so miserable that they seemed to be continually depressed and unhappy. Only you know if you are happy or unhappy with the shape of your body and with the shape of your life.

Do you believe losing weight will allow you to have a super show business career? It could. Who knows? Maybe you do have the talent to make it. Yet being thin is no guarantee of success. Fat people have done well in Hollywood. Alfred Hitchcock is certainly no lightweight, and nobody ever accused Sidney Greenstreet of being thin. That is something you have to think about and decide for yourself.

Do you think your love life will improve? Perhaps it will; perhaps it will not. After all, in some parts of the world, fat people are looked upon as very sexy. On the other hand, you may live, and probably do, in a part of the world where a thin, shapely body attracts favorable attention.

Give these questions a few minutes of deep, honest consideration. Why not put the book down and think about it for a while. Ask yourself if you really want to put out the energy and change your present point of view about eating. Because it requires that you pay attention to what you are doing. You will have to look at new ways of thinking about food, which will probably mean changing your point of view about your present eating behavior.

Let us say, just as an example, that you usually eat a quart of ice cream a day. Now, you know that to lose weight that daily quart of ice cream has to go. Maybe this is not worth the effort to you. Maybe you are not interested in learning a new behavior. Only you can make that choice.

I sincerely wish I could tell you that I have a magic wand and that when I wave it, all the unwanted fat on your body will vanish. I do not have any such thing. If I did, I would not have written a book, I would just crisscross the country and wave fat away. What I can do is to help you to help yourself.

The scale illustrated here may assist you in deciding. It is different from the one in your bathroom that you use—or do not use. It is a list of emotions or feelings felt by fat people, or Eating Losers, as I prefer to call them, versus Eating Winners, people who want to be and are thin. All the emotions are rated on a scale of 1 through 10. On the left are the negative or minus feelings; on the right are the positive or plus feelings. An emotion rated as 1 (on either the plus or minus side) is weak; an emotion rated as 10 is strong.

Look over the chart. Do you feel any of the negative emotions to some degree? Would you like to have more of the positive emotions? If so, all you have to do is learn to experience more and more of the positive feelings so you can remove the barriers standing between the "fat you" and the "thin you." Remove the barriers and there is no reason why you cannot solve the problem of your weight.

Where do you weigh-in the heaviest? On the positive side or on the negative side? Are you pleased with your emotional weigh-in? If you find yourself with a heavy negative score, would you rather develop a heavy positive score?

					Minus											Plus					
10	9	8	7	6	5	4	3	2	1	0	1	2	3	4	5	6	7	8	9	10	

Minus		Plus
Disgust	*	Gratification
Shame	*	Pleasure
Tension	*	Contentment
Anger	*	Confidence
Aggression	*	Delight
Guilt	*	Relaxation
Resentment	*	Peacefulness
Fear	*	Excitement
Frustration	*	Honesty
Irritation	*	Freedom
Discomfort	*	Joy
Insecurity	*	
Deceit	*	
Pain	*	
Negative Emotions of Eating Losers	B A R R I E R S	Positive Emotions of Eating Winners

Think about this for a while. Take as long as you want. The choice is yours. What is more important to you—eating a quart of ice cream and afterwards having a negative self-evaluation, or learning to forgo the ice cream and having a positive evaluation?

Should you decide to remove the barriers, you will be setting a goal for yourself: to create more positive feelings and to lose *x* number of pounds. Are you willing to stick to your goal? A firm commitment is necessary because that is an important part of losing weight.

Should you decide you really want to lose weight and that you are willing to stick to your goal, and should you become a successful goal achiever, I can only point out that you will have the right to say proudly, to yourself and to everybody else, "I achieved my goal of losing weight. I did a fine job." Beyond that, being happy, famous, beautiful, or successful is your responsibility. It is your life and your body, and only you have the right to make *decisions* affecting them. (It is perfectly all right if you wish to discuss your thoughts on the matter with others.)

Should you decide you are not really interested in losing weight, for whatever reason, I respect your decision. But if you truly want to lose weight, I believe I can assist you. Let's begin now.

Once you have set your goal—to lose *x* number of pounds —how will you go about achieving this goal? Will you go on a diet? There is no need for that, because you are on one already. You have been on a diet all your life.

When you read that last sentence, your reaction probably was: "You better believe I've been on a diet all my life. I don't know how many diets I've tried, and not one of them worked."

Well, at least one of them must have worked, because you are still here to read this book. Now you are thinking, "If a diet had worked for me, I wouldn't be reading this book."

Not necessarily. What is a diet anyway? Think about it. What is your answer? A diet is something to make you lose weight? Is it? Not according to the dictionary.

One of the definitions of "diet" in *Webster's New Collegiate Dictionary* is: "What a person or animal usually eats or drinks daily." So if you have been eating nothing but peanut butter and jelly sandwiches for the past twenty years, you have been on a diet: your daily fare has been peanut butter and jelly sandwiches. Whatever you have been eating all these years has been your diet. So, since you are still here, your diet has worked in that it has kept you alive.

However, if you want to lose weight, then your diet is not

working for you the way you want it to. What you are looking
for is an eating behavior or pattern that will keep you alive,
yet allow you to lose weight. This can be called a reducing
diet, but I do not particularly like the term. It conjures up
visions of something temporary: the dieter knocks off a certain number of pounds by following some low-calorie plan
for a while, then once a satisfactory weight is achieved, he
goes back to eating the way he did before the weight loss.
Most people reduce so they can get back to eating.

This is where I feel many people get off purpose on these
so-called reducing diets, and why so many "fail" on them.
Since no new behavior is learned, they run the risk of gaining back the weight they lost. They have no choice but to
continue on the reducing program or return to the old style
of eating—the fat style. It is like being caught between the
devil and the deep blue sea because they have never learned
anything other than their original eating behavior—a fat
eating behavior.

There is another choice, and that is what I want to present
to you in this book. It is learning a new eating behavior, a
thin eating behavior. Once you have learned a new behavior
—thin eating—then you can choose between an eating style
that works for your personal goals and one that does not.
Solving a weight problem is essentially a matter of learning an
eating behavior to add to your present eating habits. The first
step in learning a new, thin eating behavior is to switch from
what I call automatic pilot to manual pilot. What am I talking about?

People with a weight problem are usually not really aware
of the food they consume. This is what automatic pilot is—a
relinquishing of *conscious* control. If food is there, fat people
on automatic eat it. No choice is exercised. Reaching out for
food can be like an automatic reflex; no thought is given to
the action—especially no thoughts like, "Is eating this food
purposeful, is eating this food oriented toward my goal?"
Generally, fat people do not know, because they may not

notice what they are eating. The available choices are ignored. My eating behavior in the New York restaurant was an example of automatic pilot.

Today, when I operate on manual pilot, it is just the opposite. When operating on manual, you do not eat any food without giving it thought. I'm not talking about deep philosophical thought; just plain, ordinary, everyday consideration. You are always aware of what you are eating, how much, and what it tastes like. People who eat on manual pilot know whether the food is enjoyable and if it is purposeful. The way I was eating in the Honolulu restaurant is an example of the manual pilot style.

The awareness present when you're on manual pilot is really of eating *and* enjoying food because full attention is given to the act. When you operate on manual pilot, you learn to savor every bite of food you put in your mouth. You also give close attention to the chewing, swallowing, and digesting of the food.

But since this book is about learning, let's talk about how really easy learning can be by looking at how you and I learned to be fat.

3

Learning to Be Fat

Right now you are probably thinking, "I learned to be fat? Nonsense! Nobody ever sat me down and gave me lessons in being fat." Of course not. Nobody ever sat me down either. I never took a single lesson in being fat, but I learned anyway. So did you. And the fact that we learned to be fat only proves you can learn to be thin, just as I did.

If you still have your doubts that you learned to be fat, you might like to know how I learned. As you read this chapter, you are likely to find that your experiences have been similar to mine. Using my two scenarios (my dinners in New York and Hawaii) as a basis for comparison, we can start discussing the various aspects of learning and changing.

People do not need formal lessons to learn things. There are many ways for human beings to learn. Learning to talk is a good example. This is one of my favorite examples because I have observed the process first-hand. When my goddaughter, Raina, was learning to talk she was demonstrating a learning process. As the early weeks and months of Raina's life went by, she was surrounded by the sounds of human speech, but nobody gave her formal lessons. Then came the day when she said her first word. When this happened, her parents were very excited about it (so was I, because her

first word happened to be "Larry"). They showed their pleasure with a great deal of hugging and happy fussing.

As young as Raina was, she felt the approval of those
around her. This approval encouraged her to continue her
attempts at speech. Raina learned to talk, and this is exactly
how you and I learned to talk. There were no formal lessons;
but one day, our noises became words. Feeling the approval,
we learned more phrases, and soon we were building words
into sentences. Many of us learned to be fat in a similar way.

People who know a lot about learning seem to think that
there are primarily three modes that influence the way we
learn. Often these modes work in conjunction with each
other.

The Operant Mode: This form of learning received a great
deal of publicity as a result of the work done by Dr. B. F.
Skinner of Harvard University. Essentially, this mode involves a system of rewards and punishments to shape behavior. Skinner's experiments made use of pigeons. The
pigeons learned that they would be rewarded with food
if they manipulated a lever with their beaks. Pigeons not
pecking at the lever were punished with an absence of food.
The conclusion is that people behave as they do as a result
of the consequences of their behavior. This is the scholarly
view of the theory; there are those who claim the pigeons
see it differently. Supposedly one pigeon was overheard saying to another, "Watch how well I've trained this guy. Every
time I peck at the lever, he feeds me."

Although Dr. Skinner's work generated controversy, the
Operant Mode has been in use for years; grandmothers have
been rewarding their grandchildren with cookies long before
B. F. Skinner, and for all anyone knows, a Stone Age mother
may have used this form of learning. If a child does something which is considered to be good, like saying a word,
someone rewards the behavior—there is a great deal of hugging, smiling, and praising. This emotional reward encour-
ages the child to say another word—or at least the child

knows what he has done is acceptable and that people are pleased. Conversely, if the child does something unacceptable, such as telling a lie, a punishment follows—perhaps a whack on the backside. From this, the child learns the unpleasant consequences of lying.

This punishment aspect, or adverse conditioning, as it is also called, was dramatically portrayed in Stanley Kubrick's movie *A Clockwork Orange*. Adverse conditioning, when it works, serves only to stop a behavior, positive or pleasant. Alternatives are usually not offered.

The Operant Mode can also teach us ways to avoid food. My mother does not care for tomatoes and avoids eating them whenever she can by saying she is allergic to them. Mom has no such allergy, but she learned that this is an acceptable excuse for not eating them. Rather than saying, "I don't like tomatoes," and hearing, "But tomatoes are good for you," or some such thing, Mom found out that when people are told, "I break out in a rash from tomatoes," the subject is dropped. Many people learn the same little tricks to avoid certain foods. One explanation, whether accurate or not, produces better results than another.

Another example of the Operant Mode is using food so it becomes a reward. The little kid who comes dashing home from school with a great report card and is told by his proud mother, "Why, that's wonderful! You've earned an ice cream sundae," is learning to expect food for acceptable behavior. Good report cards can well become the norm if ice cream sundaes are offered as a reward—of course the result could also be a fat kid.

Fatness can also be taught by adverse conditioning. The old ploy of many an exasperated mother, "If you don't stop crying right now, you'll go to bed without supper!" is an example. The kid soon learns to behave so he can eat.

Arousing a sense of guilt is also part of adverse conditioning. Nobody I've ever met enjoys feeling guilty about something. A feeling of guilt is often introduced to make a child eat unwanted food. Usually instilling a sense of guilt works because the emotion is unpleasant. Another emotion that can be used is fear—fear that there will be no food at some future date or that too little food in the present will cause illness in the future.

Both emotions, guilt and fear, are brought to bear in what has become a familiar plaint in many American homes: "Clean your plate." We have all been exposed to the "Clean plate club" ploy at one time or another. It goes like this: "Eat all your carrots so you won't get a lot of colds in the winter." Or, "How can you leave food on your plate when the starving Armenians would love to have it?" When I was a kid I heard a lot about the Starving Armenians, though I had no idea of what an Armenian was. I did, though, have visions of poor, skinny people grubbing around in garbage pails looking for food. Ironically, the first Armenian I did meet was most corpulent and ate heroic meals.

The Classical Mode: Don't let the name throw you. This mode of learning refers to the work done by the Russian scientist Ivan Pavlov. His experiment involved a dog, meat powder, and a bell. Each time Pavlov gave the dog meat powder, he rang a bell. Whenever the dog was given the meat powder, he would salivate. After a while, all Pavlov had to do was ring the bell and the dog would salivate.

We learn to associate food with certain events in exactly the same way. If every time Grandma visits, she brings a box of cookies, a little kid is going to learn to associate her visits with food. Once this happens, all that is necessary is an announcement, "Grandma is coming this afternoon," and the child is all set for cookies. But the Classical Mode does not always require a physical stimulus. Emotions as well as sounds, sights, smells, and events can trigger a similar response. Many people overeat when experiencing certain feelings like anger, pain, or depression; it is their way of reacting to stress.

Modeling: I agree with Dr. Albert Bandura of Stanford University that imitation is probably the most powerful form of learning, and that we all use this method. What makes it particularly powerful is the fact that we use modeling all of our lives.

Modeling (or vicarious learning) is copying the behavior of another. Sometimes we deliberately imitate the behavior of a person we admire; at other times we are unaware of our imitative behavior. How many times have you heard statements like, "Stuart is the spitting image of his father; he even has the same gestures"? Whether he is aware of it or not, Stuart has learned to model his behavior on his father's.

The same goes for food. We see our parents eating a certain way, and we copy their behavior. If our parents make a point of scraping their plates at every meal, so do we. If our parents rush through meals, so do we. By modeling my eating behavior on my mother's, for example, I picked up her aversion for tomatoes. For a long time I was wary of tomatoes, which brings up my next point.

Modeling has one disadvantage. It is not always purposeful. It can be random with no thought given to whether the model is a negative or positive influence.

One, two, or all three modes can be employed in teaching someone to be fat. Obviously, as in most everyone's case, all three modes probably played a part in my learning to be fat.

When I was a kid growing up in Mount Vernon, New York, my family always ate dinner at six o'clock, and I was expected to be at the table. Whether or not I was hungry did not seem to be a factor. Dinner was at a specific time, and I soon got the message that if I didn't appear I brought down the stern displeasure of my parents. My mother wanted to fix one meal per evening and get done in the kitchen. So every evening, promptly at six o'clock, I parked myself at the table and ate. This behavior made everybody happy—my parents were happy because I was learning to cooperate within the structure of the family; I was happy because my parents were happy even though there were times when I wanted to be out playing stickball with my friends.

From this came a sort of underlying belief that *eating had nothing to do with hunger*. Eating had to do with food being put in front of me. Eating was not something to do because I wanted to; rather it was something to do because the clock said it was time.

Furthermore, no time was lost in initiating me into the Clean Plate Club. Wasting food was an awful thing in my family. Mom rarely, if ever, threw food away. If she or I didn't want the leftovers, Dad would take them, saying, "No sense in letting good food go to waste."

Whatever the reason for joining the Clean Plate Club— guilt, parental example, or some belief in the curative powers of food—we can easily become lifetime members. When I pulled the châteaubriand snatch in the New York restaurant, I was still an executive board member in very good standing. And with this attitude toward food, I most certainly was not going to let a dessert go to waste!

Learning to be fat also involves living up to expectations. Other people expect us to exhibit certain behavior, and we come across with the expected behavior to oblige them.

When I was a young boy, I was crazy about milk; when I was in the mood, I could drink almost a gallon at one sitting —I kid you not. This ability attracted a lot of attention. Why not? It was unusual behavior. I also had a very close friend who lived not too far away. Every time I went to see my friend and ate dinner at his house, his mother, Edie, would have at least three quarts of milk in the refrigerator. As I walked into the house, she always greeted me with, "There's plenty of milk here for you, Larry. I knew you were coming this evening, so I bought a few extra quarts."

Well, what could I do? I had no other choice; no other learned behavior to choose from. Edie had been thoughtful enough to buy extra milk for me, so I showed my appreciation for her concern by drinking it. I never thought about whether I wanted the milk or not; I liked to think I was an extremely polite guest. I drank it all. That is what we learn. Don't be rude and hurt people's feelings by refusing the food they offer you! Show your appreciation and eat.

We also learn to be fat because we live where we do. America is a bountiful country. Having enough food has never been much of a problem for most of us. However, having enough food to eat often means eating a lot of food. Big, heaping servings. None of this "a dab of this and a dash of that." Shovel it on the plate! Why skimp when we can enjoy as much as we want as often as we want? My parents were never stingy about food, and chances are, yours were not either. So as our mothers heaped our plates at mealtime, many of us absorbed the implicit message that food was to be eaten in quantity, the larger the better.

Along with all my other lessons, I also found out what food could do if I was bored, angry, or depressed about something. All of this is probably familiar to you, and similar lessons probably produced similar results. Before much time had gone by, you and I learned that eating food had nothing to do with being hungry. Food was not to be ignored —it was to be consumed, and quickly. Put food in front of us, and we would dig right in. We had learned to be on automatic pilot.

And was I ever on automatic pilot! By not controlling my eating habits, I got heavier and heavier. I went from a chubby eight-year-old to a just plain fat twenty-eight-year-old. I even worked myself into some very embarrassing situations.

One evening while I was still a resident on the gynecological service, a nurse stopped me as she was going to dinner to ask me a question about a patient. Putting her sandwich and an open bag of potato chips down on the desk, she pulled the chart, and I answered her question. Not wanting to keep her from her dinner, I said, "Enjoy your dinner." To my surprise, she answered my pleasantry in an icy voice: "I had hoped to, Doctor, but you just ate part of it." That was news to me, but

I looked. Sure enough, as we stood discussing the patient for those few minutes, I had devoured most of her remaining potato chips.

One glance at her face told me that my stammered apologies and my offer to buy another bag of potato chips were not going to restore me to her good graces that fast.

As I write about this incident now, it is funny; but believe me, it was not funny at the time. I felt really foolish, and I also knew that the story would be told and retold in the nurses' lounge until it became part of the hospital legend. For weeks I was convinced that everyone, even the patients, were laughing about it.

Even Ron Pion's kids were caught by my eating behavior. Ron's wife, Gail, maintains a cookie jar well stocked with one of my favorite snacks—chocolate chip cookies. Gail makes the cookies for Jeff, Dana, and Tracy Pion; but there was a time when I was eating more than the three kids put together. Every time I visited the Pions, I headed straight for the cookie jar. It became something of a joke with the kids. Whenever Gail told them I was coming, they'd say, "Hide the cookies."

Boredom also kept me munching away. After that dinner in New York, I wandered into the coffee shop because I had nothing else to do, or so I believed. Similar situations would occasionally arise at the hospital. A few years back, many of the prime time television shows had a hospital motif. You probably remember these programs. They were called "The Doctors," "The Nurses," "The Interns," "The Orderlies," or some such title. Just about every facet of the medical profession had a television program of its own. Every once in a while I would watch these shows and be intrigued by the way the scriptwriters saw hospital life. The opening scenes always had hospital personnel rushing around pushing stretchers or dashing off with an intravenous bottle or a pint of blood. And the story itself always involved some highly unlikely but dramatic situation: a nurse has a nervous breakdown in the operating room right in the middle of tricky brain surgery and tries to kill the chief surgeon with a scalpel. Obviously some of the plots were really far out, and I watched the shows just for laughs, or perhaps excitement, because hospital routine is rarely like it is pictured on the television screen.

Sometimes a work shift in a hospital can be quiet and peaceful. Even downright boring, especially if you expect a lot of dashing around. I found this out during the times I was on night duty in one of the slower maternity wards. Perhaps a few deliveries would occur, but no emergencies to speak of; and with nothing to do but kill time, I would wander down to the nurses' station and have coffee and something to eat with them. Patients are always giving the nurses gifts of food like candy or cookies, so there was usually something for me to munch on.

At one Honolulu hospital, I especially enjoyed being with the nurses on the 11 to 7 shift. Not only were they great people, but they also brought in terrific Oriental goodies to nibble on. Or I would corner a colleague and eat with him. It did not matter who I was with or what I was eating, just so long as time passed. That was the important thing. I had yet to learn how to become excited with myself and to create that excitement from within me. I expected my external environment to do it for me.

My particular hang-up was boredom; it could be yours, too. There can be others. Many shy, fat people hide their self-consciousness in a social situation by eating. Shoveling food into their mouths gives them something to do with their hands. A number of lonely people view food as companionship; as long as they have food, they have something (rather than someone) to keep them company. I also know people who use food to smother their anger. Whenever they feel they are about to lose their temper, no matter how justified they may be, they turn to food to calm them down.

In the end, the lessons have been well learned. You and I

became Masters of Miseating, and as a consequence, we were overweight. We have proved our ability to miseat to ourselves and to the world many times over. However, once I learned to be fat, then I moved on to the next thing, as you have. I learned to stay fat. I built my barriers and became a prisoner of my past.

4

Staying Fat

Every now and again when I meet someone with a weight problem our conversation will get around to the subject of losing weight. I may hear things like, "If I stopped eating salted peanuts maybe I'd lose weight, but I can't. I've got this thing about salted peanuts." I might answer this statement with something like, "When I was fat, my hang-up was chocolate chip cookies." A remark like this can bring forth a surprised, "You were fat? You of all people—a doctor! I'd think you'd know better."

Of course I knew better, but my past learning worked against it. Doctors are subject to learning principles, too. They have the same strengths, weaknesses, and foibles as other people. I know quite a few doctors who have to be dragged kicking and screaming to see a dentist just like a lot of other people. Despite the evidence that smoking is a dangerous habit, many doctors smoke. What a person does for a living is no guarantee of being either fat or thin. How a person thinks, feels, and acts about himself is what determines success or failure in any endeavor.

Once I had become a Master of Miseating and had allowed myself to run on automatic pilot, it seemed as if I had no choice. I could only continue as I was, since I did not know how to change my eating habits and lose weight. I continued on automatic pilot. To ensure this continued behavior, I built many barriers and became a prisoner of my past. I did not allow myself the option of learning a new way to be. I only behaved as I had learned to be in my past.

To do this, I did not lie to myself (or anybody else). I told the truth—as I saw it. I was not fat. I was big-boned and broad-shouldered. I was a big, hefty football player. I got a lot of mileage out of that one. My football career was brief— I never really enjoyed the game, so I stopped playing. But long after my football "career" ended, I was trotting that excuse out of the closet.

When I was not using football as a brick to build my prison of fat, I was claiming that I needed all that food to stay in tip-top shape. As a doctor, I could not run the risk of becoming shaky or dizzy or weak. "What would happen," I asked myself, "if I got a case of the shakes while performing an operation or delivering a baby? I cannot take a chance like that. I would be violating my oath as a doctor!" This line of reasoning was one of my favorites because it made me feel good about my motives, even virtuous. Actually it was sanctimonious nonsense, and I know that now.

Two bricks do not a prison make. There were other excuses. Whenever I entertained at my place, there was usually a lot of food left over. No matter how many people I invited, they always ate far less than I served. After my guests had gone, I would start munching away at the remainders, and then munch a little more as I told myself, "The food will just go to waste even if I put it in the refrigerator, since I'll be on call at the hospital for the next thirty-six hours. Waste not, want not, as Grandmother used to say." Even when I knew full well that the food would not spoil if refrigerated for a day or two, I still told myself that I did not want to take the chance. It was easier to eat the food than figure out how to store it. This behavior was something else that made me feel good. I was not wasting food.

Another thing that kept me behind a barrier of fat was the

fact that my three hundred pounds did not seem to be a problem. I was a successful person, I had friends. I was a good student. I had no trouble getting into medical school. I liked the way my career was going. People liked me. I had a terrific relationship with a beautiful, intelligent woman named Michelle.

The work that Ron and I were doing was getting favorable attention. I was being noticed and acknowledged for my research. In 1971, Ortho Pharmaceutical Corporation awarded me their first Ortho Fellowship in Family Planning and Human Sexuality. And in 1972 I got the opportunity to do ob-gyn research in Uganda with Sultan Karim, a leading pharmacologist who was doing exciting work with a new reproductive drug. I had assets—my life was a positive experience. "You can't have everything," I reasoned. "What more could a man want, so why worry about a few extra pounds?" That is, if I ever thought about my weight, which I did not do very often. After all, I was really a big, husky football player.

My behavior in the New York coffee shop was another example of learned behavior that allowed me to eat. Beyond buying the magazine, there was no excuse for what I was doing. The chair in my room was uncomfortable. Oh, sure. Yet there were very comfortable chairs in the lobby, and as a guest of the hotel I had every right to make use of them. I chose the coffee shop, where I could order food. I knew then that coffee shops are not reading rooms, yet I set myself up. Once inside, I could do nothing else, or so I reasoned, but eat. I had no choice, really, since I had not yet learned a different eating behavior.

As I write this chapter and glance back over what I have written, I find that I cannot even claim my rationalizations were particularly original. I was using the same type of bricks to build a wall to encase myself in fat that everybody else uses. Oh, maybe there were variations in size and color, but the bricks were bricks and the result was the same.

And the same result is always achieved no matter what the reasoning. Many overweight people fall back on the excuse that they have "big bones." Broad shoulders and broad hips have been blamed for the excess poundage from years of overeating. Genes are also blamed for fat. A goodly number of people I work with tell me, "Fat runs in my family. I inherited this tendency to gain weight. I must have. My mother and father are both fat." Fat people tend to come from fat families because the whole family overeats together, and they learn from each other. Red hair and green eyes may be inherited in your family, but fat is not. You simply do not inherit fat.

Another popular rationalization for fat is some physical disorder beyond the individual's control. After I lost weight, a man I know slightly stopped me in a grocery store one morning and congratulated me on my loss, adding, "I wish I could knock off about fifty or sixty pounds, but I can't. I've got this thyroid condition . . . " Well, if it is not a thyroid disorder, then it is a low rate of basal metabolism—anything but eating too much food. Blaming a physical condition for obesity is a way of not taking responsibility—since only you can change the way you are.

Yet all these excuses and rationalizations are perfectly understandable. No one likes to admit, "It's my own fault that I'm fat. I have put my eating behavior on automatic pilot and have forgotten about it." I know I did not want to admit it, either to myself or to anybody else.

Perhaps the brick that was most firmly implanted in my barrier wall of fat was the one allowing me to believe that my past was the best indicator of my future. I had always been overweight; therefore, I would always be so. My weight was something I had no control over. Why fight the inevitable? I decided that if I was meant to weigh three hundred pounds, then I would weigh three hundred pounds. It did not strike me as the worst thing in the world. So, based on my past, I settled for a fat future. That was a mistake I made, and I want to assist you in avoiding a similar error. If you have already made that error, I want to show you that you can correct it. You can change your present behavior starting right now.

The past is a funny thing. It is an excellent tool if we use it properly; it is a machine out of control if we abuse it. The past is an excellent servant if we let it serve us; it is a tyrant if we allow ourselves to serve it. This may strike you as an unnecessarily philosophical statement to find in a book about losing weight and keeping it off. It really isn't, because far too many heavy people allow themselves to be chained to their past. They allow their past to tyrannize them and to dictate their present and future behavior.

Having been overweight for a number of years, many people falsely assume they always will be. When this happens, the past becomes a prison. It was, therefore it will be. So many people, when I first meet them, have a low self-image because of their weight and doubt their ability to solve their weight problem. They make defeatist statements like, "I don't know why I'm wasting my time and yours by talking about this. I've always been fat, and I know I always will be."

This belief is all too familiar. After all, I subscribed to it myself. When I was seven or eight, I started to pack on the pounds. Once the weight had been around for over twenty years, I assumed it would be there for another twenty. I had become a servant of my past, and people who say "I've always been fat" are victims of the same tyranny.

If you mistakenly believe that because you were fat twelve months ago you will be fat twelve months from now, let me ask you the same question I ask other people who feel this way: Did you always know how to tie your shoes? Whenever I ask this question, I usually get a look as though I am out of my mind. Right now, you are probably thinking the same thing. No, I am not out of my mind, I am very serious. Did you always know how to tie your shoes? Your answer has to be no, because shoe tying is a skill we learned a few years after we were born. No one, not even a genius, is born with this skill. It has to be learned, acquired. Once that skill is no longer used, perhaps because of an injury or a disease like arthritis, we really appreciate what a useful skill it is and how little attention we paid to it.

What this is leading up to is that at some time in our past, we lacked a skill we have today. Just because there was a time when we could not tie our shoes by ourselves did not mean we had to live our entire lives without this skill. The past can be a very inaccurate gauge of the future. However, the past can be a very accurate prediction of the future, especially when it works for you; that is, when your goals are being met. If this is not so, then the past is, as I said, an inaccurate gauge of the future. The fact that you were fat twelve months ago means nothing. Last year is gone, behind you, and there is nothing to change it. Clinging to the past, serving the past when it is not working for you, makes as much sense as saying, "Because I knocked a glass off the table and broke it last Wednesday, I will break a glass this coming Wednesday, and every future Wednesday."

The present and the future are the important frameworks. What you think, feel, and do about yourself are of the utmost importance. You can start learning to eat "thinner" today so you will be thinner next month. As far as I know, it is impossible to reshape the past. But it is so easy to shape the future!

The past can tyrannize us in another way. Many times people say to me, "I just can't lose weight. I know, because I've tried before. If I had a dollar for every time I tried a reducing plan, I'd be rich. Nothing ever worked for me. I failed at them all."

Having tried reducing plans in the past means nothing, absolutely nothing. So what if you tried to follow a plan and could not stick it out long enough for results to show? How long did you follow the plan? A week? A month? Five months? Do not give it any thought. In my opinion, it seems that the popular reducing schemes are not designed for success. They are boring and usually require you to follow some complicated measuring or counting formula. The person who has not lost weight using one of these plans has not failed; rather he has decided the results were not worth the effort involved. And the results are not worth the effort, because there is an easier way to lose weight.

The so-called failures you may have experienced with these programs prove nothing except that you do not like drinking eight glasses of water a day, or that you want more variety than grapefruit offers, or that you find toting a postal scale around with you a nuisance. What you have established, indeed learned, is that time-consuming weight-loss programs do not appeal to you.

Then what *do* we do with the past? Absolutely nothing. Leave it alone. It is over and done with. All you have to do is put the past to one side. Put the past in the attic of your mind where you store all the other information you no longer use.

Kicking yourself, punishing yourself, criticizing yourself will change nothing. There is no need to waste time trying when you can use your energies in more positive and purposeful activities. After all, the future lies ahead, and all you need do is use it well. If the past is working for you—terrific. If it is not, leave it alone, and let's get excited about learning a new behavior. But remember: only if you want to.

5

The Great Escape

Whenever people learn that I was once fat, they ask, "What made you decide to lose weight?" It is a fair question and a logical one; but frankly, it is a question that I am hard pressed to answer. There was no great revelation. I cannot claim that one day I girded my loins and went forth to do battle against the fat of Larry Reich. When I knew I would write a book describing my weight loss and learning to be thin, I gave a lot of thought to the question of just what started me toward the goal of being thin. In the end, I realized my decision to learn a new eating behavior was the result of several things that took place over a period of time.

I do know what was not the cause. Many people assumed, inaccurately, that I lost weight because Michelle would not date me when I was heavy. Other people jumped to the conclusion that Michelle had convinced me to reduce. Neither is the case. Michelle and I were already seeing each other before I started to lose weight. Furthermore, Michelle had always been interested in me as an individual. She accepted me as a heavy person in very much the same way she accepts me as a thin person today. That is not to imply that changes in the physical and emotional environment have not altered our lives. In fact they have, and the nice thing about it is that we have grown—in very positive ways. Michelle and I have both grown and benefited by the experience.

After I lost all my fat, though, I asked for her candid opinion of the new me, and if the old me had ever bothered her. "Now that I have a basis for comparison," she told me, "I think you're a more attractive man since you've lost weight, and I'm proud of your success. But when we first met, I never thought of you as fat or thin—you were Larry." While Michelle had nothing to do with the initial decision, she did, however, support me every inch of the way.

If I had to pick out a starting point for my transformation, it would be my involvement in est training. As a result of est, I became aware that there was a lot of boredom in my life. I also noticed the two periods in my life when I had gained the most weight. One was when I was in medical school, and the other had been during my residency. During both periods I was very bored. Life seemed to lack excitement and challenge, and I ate too much.

Conversely, I noticed that during one of the most eventful periods of my life I had lost weight. That was during my stay in Uganda in 1972. Originally I had gone there to become involved in some exciting research with a new drug that seemed to have a possible use in reproductive health. From the very first, Uganda proved stimulating: the physicians and scientists I met, the research being done, and just the idea of living in a different cultural environment. My stay, however, turned out to be even more exciting than I had anticipated.

While there, I was caught in the expulsion of Asians that was ordered by Uganda's now infamous President Idi Amin Dada. Most of the friends I had made and lived with were Indians who did not support him, and they asked me to help get their belongings out of the country. For several weeks I was smuggling money, jewelry, documents, and medicines out of Uganda. Talk about exciting! Boredom was a feeling I had no time for.

My smuggling activities stopped when I was arrested. While sitting in a jail cell, hungry as I was, I had other things on my mind besides food. Thoughts like: Would I get out alive? Whenever the door was unlocked, I did not think, "Maybe the guard is bringing me food." It was more like, "Maybe it's my turn to be shot." Not surprisingly, my reduced food intake, combined with the anxiety, meant I lost some weight.

Well, there was one answer—right in front of me. Boredom meant eating too much and being fat. Excitement and stimulation (not to mention fear) meant eating less and losing weight. I was able to lose weight! I did not have to be fat!

During est I also reaffirmed that the work I was doing with Ron Pion was exciting and challenging, but I had never channeled the excitement toward losing weight before. So there was another answer. All I had to do was notice the excitement and challenges already present in my life and create more. From this I saw I had always had two paths open to me—the negative one called boredom which did not work for me and the positive one called enthusiasm which did work for me. And I knew how to use both. It was up to me to choose which outlook I wanted for my life.

I opted to do something about my feelings of ennui. What I did was pick myself up and move. I went looking for new interests and activities while at the same time noticing what was challenging about my life already. I found them, too. Suddenly, instead of looking for ways to "kill" time by eating, there was a new problem confronting me—how to find enough time in each day to do all the things I wanted to do! With so many things to do, I was eating less. As a result of less food, I began to lose weight—not a remarkable amount at first, but enough pounds slipped off to make me realize that losing weight wasn't such a hard thing after all. I was not *destined* to be fat, and I did not need all that food I had been shoving into my mouth! I had proof that I would not get dizzy, faint, or exhausted if my food intake was reduced.

While est helped me to clarify my life-style goals and therefore played a part in my weight loss, I was, of course, influenced by other things. My interest in clothing, especially European designs, played a part. Yet I rarely bought anything—because I rarely found anything that fit me. Occasionally, while shopping in New York I found a designer suit that fit, and this discovery would fill me with glee. Living in Honolulu, however, gave me a terrific excuse to ignore my interest in clothing.

I would tell myself that dress in the Islands was so informal that I would never wear a designer suit. Furthermore, all I really needed were hospital scrub suits. Of course scrub suits, size XXL, were all that fit me. The day finally came when even an XXL was tight. Not that I saw it as my problem. The scrub suit, I decided, had been poorly made or perhaps mismarked.

Michelle, however, is deeply involved in the fashion world. She knows a great deal about it, and as we got to know each other better, my dormant interest in clothing came to life again. I wanted to be able to buy clothes—designer clothes—whenever I felt like it. There was only one way I could do it: I had to lose weight. Whether I liked it or not, the men's clothing industry does not cater to the three-hundred-pound male any more than the world's fashion centers cater to the three-hundred-pound woman.

There were probably other things that helped me reach my decision to lose weight, but these are the things that stand out in my mind. Least of all was the fact that I was a very successful person and the fear of failing at losing weight was something I hadn't been ready to confront until then.

Along with knowing I could survive very well on less food and that by eating less food I could lose weight, there was other important information available to me—I knew a lot about learning and how people learn. We are what we are because of what we learned. I was fat because I had learned to eat that way; therefore, it seemed reasonable that I could also learn to eat in a way that would allow me to be thin.

There was something else I knew a great deal about, and that was problem-solving. In fact, assisting people in learning to solve their problems had become of great interest to me, since my chosen career was helping people solve problems related to sex and reproduction. At first, though, I did not realize that the problem-solving techniques that I had applied to my own weight loss could be used by others.

In fact, after I achieved my weight goal, people with weight problems began to call me, and I explained that assisting with a weight problem was not my area. Then Ron and I started exploring the question of weight loss. We had known for some time that the formation of problems and their solutions had very similar characteristics regardless of the problem itself. We form all our problems in much the same way. Whatever is troubling people—sex, alcohol, tobacco, weight—the problem can be handled in the same way. Consequently, the people we see every week are troubled by just about every possible human problem, including weight. My advice worked for me, it has worked for others, and I believe it will work for you!

6

Choices, Choices All Around

To lose weight or not to lose weight is your choice; only you can make that decision. And by "only you," I mean just that. Nobody else can choose for you—not your spouse, or your best friend, or your parents. Being responsible implies being able to respond to your own wants and needs. Before we start talking about choice and what it means in our lives, let's go back to the dictionary for a moment for a precise definition of the word. Webster's defines choice as: A choosing; selection; the right or power to choose; option. Further on, we read that choice "implies the chance, right, or power to choose, usually by the free exercise of one's judgment."

Think about that and how it applies to your life. For many people, this is a particularly troublesome concept. "What? Me make a choice? I can hardly decide what to wear in the morning." How often have I heard that or some similar remark! You might feel that way yourself. Making a choice is almost impossible, out of the question, you cannot do it. Is that so?

Well, unless you are reading this book in a prison library, you do make choices in your life. You do decide eventually what you will wear every morning. Maybe you do not like to make choices, maybe it takes a while; but still, in the end, you do make them. Choice implies responsibility, and many people, I know, seem to do whatever they can to avoid taking responsibility—especially for their behavior. Yet even when some people sidestep responsibility, they are, in reality, choosing—to sidestep the issue.

Everybody, even little kids, decides things. Maybe you do not see it that way, but even kids make choices. Have you ever watched a child with a coloring book and an assortment of crayons? Each time he or she picks up a yellow crayon when it could just as easily have been a blue one, a choice has been made. Choosing a crayon may not strike you as the most earth-shattering decision, but the child is learning something about making selections.

Adults who swear up and down that they cannot make choices make them all the time. Deciding to watch one television program over another is a choice. Deciding to call or not to call a friend is a choice. Deciding to lose weight or to stay heavy is a choice.

Occasionally people feel there is no choice available to them. Someone who takes the bus to work every morning may do so believing there is no other option. Yet there could be other ways that have gone unnoticed: a car, a train, a subway, a walk. The same is true for eating behavior. Many people put themselves on automatic pilot because they do not realize there is an alternative eating behavior.

No great amount of thought is given to turning on a television set or to calling a friend. No great amount of thought is given to eating or to not eating. Decision-making becomes so automatic that thought is no longer given to the alternatives. In some respects, people who seem "to take forever to make up their minds" are better off. They are investigating all possibilities, all alternatives.

There are always alternatives. One alternative to being fat is being thin. One alternative to gaining weight is losing weight. One alternative to automatic pilot is manual pilot. One alternative to being in an eating pattern that is not working for you is to form a new creative pattern that will work. All of this is a way of saying that you do not have to be the way you are if you're not pleased with it.

There is no reason for you to weigh what you do now unless you want to. We all know the usual excuses for being overweight. But your genes have not made you fat, and they will not keep you fat. Your pregnancies have not made you fat. Just because you have been overweight for the past twenty years does not mean you have to be fat for the next twenty years or even the next twenty months.

The choice is yours and only yours. If you decide you are not satisfied with yourself as you are now, it may be time to exercise your option of *not* being fat. Do keep remembering, though, that *you* decide for yourself if you like what you see. What if others have been after you about your shape? If you agree 100 percent with someone else's opinion, fine! If you like what you see, that is your business and nobody else's. Just keep in mind that if you are dissatisfied with your weight, there is an alternative.

What is probably true for many people is that they have not yet *learned* a new way to eat that allows them to lose weight and to be thin. You will never know unless you try it. Now is the time to take a long, hard look at yourself in a mirror. Do you like what you see? Are you satisfied with your body? Do you think you could look better and have a better figure?

Let us assume you do not like what you see and that you are dissatisfied with your body to the point where you want to do something about it. You have decided you want a better figure. That being the case, you are now getting ready to make a choice. Let's see what happens if your reaction is, "Okay, I'm not too thrilled with what I see in the mirror. In fact, I hate it; but I'll think about it tomorrow. Maybe tomorrow I'll start."

What you have actually done is decide—you have made a choice. Your choice is to continue as you are for at least twenty-four hours—sort of a holding pattern. See, I told you, we are always making choices, even though we have not yet learned to pay attention to them.

If you decide you are going to opt for the alternative of losing weight and being thin, that is fine. You know that your current eating behavior is not working for you. If it was, you would not have a weight problem. *What*ever you have been eating is not doing what you want it to. *How* you have been eating is not working either.

Once you make the choice to be thin, you are ready to learn a new behavior and effect change. Earlier I mentioned change, and I want to talk about it again. For so many people, the whole topic is so scary (and may even be threatening) that a few more words won't hurt. Most of us are unprepared for major changes in our lives. However, like choices, changes occur all the time, and we hardly ever notice them. If it seems easier and less difficult, we tend to continue what we are doing, even if it is not working. Change to many individuals implies the unknown and the uncertain.

Consequently, many people might hold on to their fat (and their long-time eating patterns) not because they are pleased with themselves but because they are not sure they want to change. They have not learned what change can mean to their lives, how easy it is, once they realize they are changing all the time anyway.

Some people when confronted with changing from fat to thin wonder if it is really worth it. Will their spouses still love them? Will their lives become too uncertain? Perhaps too different? Yes, change can prove sort of scary to some people—and the truth is that it need not be. Being uncomfortable with change often results in a negative attitude that closes the door to positive, purposeful change. Here is another question that might be worth considering: What is to be gained if you are sunk in unhappiness and dissatisfaction when all you have to do is turn those thoughts, feelings, and actions around to happiness and satisfaction?

Fortunately, when it comes to changing from fat to thin, you face a two-way street. If you decide the old eating behavior pleases you more than the new one, you can always go back. The changes I am talking about here—changes in your eating behavior—are not permanent unless you wish to make them so.

Let's take another look at the scale of emotions on page 15, which can assist you in making your choice. You can learn to give up the feelings associated with −10 to 0 just by leaving them alone, but when this happens, you move yourself only as far as 0 on the scale. Zero is neutral—it is the absence of dissatisfaction. It is not the presence of satisfaction. As you move from the minus numbers to 0, what you end up with is a neutral balance. One purpose of learning might be to gain something—and it could be all the positive things on the other side of the asterisk. Those asterisks represent all the barriers you have erected to keep yourself trapped in the past or stalled in neutral. Removing the barrier involves nothing more complicated than learning and changing.

So, where would you rather be—on the side with all the negative emotions like misery, or on the side with all the positive emotions like happiness? The choice is yours!

7

Your Trusted Other

Sharing our feelings, our hopes, our points of view with others can be a very enhancing aspect of living when it's done in a purposeful way. By purposeful sharing, I mean taking responsibility for what you share of yourself with others. It is not purposeful or fair to use another person as an emotional dumping ground.

Many people rarely share their goals, hopes, and beliefs with others. Usually these people keep things to themselves because they are afraid of failure or rejection. Their reasoning may go something like this: "If nobody knows I'm aiming for a promotion, then if it doesn't come through, nobody need know I didn't make the grade." Or: "If I don't ask anybody for anything, I'll never be told no."

Sometimes people who refuse to admit they want to lose weight and slim down may be thinking along the same lines. They could also be trying to protect themselves. Those with a long history of reducing attempts may deny another one so they won't hear, "What, again? You've tried so often, and you get nowhere. Why bother?" Another reason could be (and often is) to avoid temptation. If no one knows about your reducing program, you won't hear, "A little bit of dessert won't hurt you. Just this once, for me."

Then there are those who go to the opposite extreme and buttonhole people constantly to talk about their weight loss program. That is the way I was. I don't think there was a doctor, nurse, or other staff member at Kapiolani Hospital who did not know I was losing weight. The trouble was that some people were less interested in what I was doing than others—simply because I matter more to some than to others. Not everyone was interested in my achievements to the same degree. More than once, my bubbly announcement of another one-pound loss would be greeted with a neutral "That's nice," or "Good for you." I was so thrilled about my success that I was beginning to bore people, yet I could not keep my happiness to myself.

No matter what type of personality you are, from loner to gregarious, losing weight can be easier and more enjoyable if you have what I call a Trusted Other. A Trusted Other is someone (or even several people) with whom you are unusually close. A Trusted Other could be your spouse, a close relative, your best friend—anyone who supports you, who is willing to help you toward your expressed goal. A Trusted Other is someone you can be with in complete comfort—someone to whom you can confide your hopes, your fears, your desires. This can be the person you turn to when you want a good laugh or a good cry.

When you are losing weight, your Trusted Other can be there to cheer you on with each success or to help you up if you become discouraged. No matter how much you want to lose weight, there are going to be times when you may go back on automatic pilot and become discouraged. This is the time to be with your Trusted Other and share your feelings of frustration or fears of failure.

As the pounds melt away, you can share your joy and success with someone who wants you to achieve your goal. But however much you want to share with others, don't forget to share your successes with yourself.

One of the first things to consider is who you will enlist to

48 FROM FAT TO SKINNY

assist and support you. You can also consider having Trusted
Others for the different aspects of your life. Perhaps there is
someone at home and another at work or your club you want
to share with. Then issue the invitation. Explain very clearly
that you are looking for support as well as for someone to
share with. A Trusted Other can, but does not have to, experiment with you. The two of you can learn together how to
prepare "new" foods like fruits and vegetables. There are
many, many ways of preparing salads to make them mouth-
watering. You and your Trusted Other can find the ways
together.

Another way your Trusted Other can assist you is by giving you suggestions. Little things like, "Do you really want
to put two sugars in your coffee?" or, "Won't that food be
just as nourishing without the butter?" It goes without saying
that your Trusted Other is not supposed to be a jailer or an
overseer, just a warm, loving, and helping friend.

In my case Michelle and Ron Pion served as my Trusted
Others. When I decided I was going to lose weight, they were
the first people I discussed my plans with, and both agreed to
support me 100 percent. Michelle is a super cook, a real
whiz at whipping up gourmet feasts. She and I decided to
turn her talents to discovering how many delicious ways we
could prepare a raw zucchini or carrot. We soon turned the
whole thing into a game. Each pound gone was as much a
joy to her as it was to me.

Being with Michelle meant I could relax completely, because I knew she would never try to slip me a piece of pecan
pie and justify her action by telling me she made the pastry
just for me. And Ron got so caught up with what I was doing
that he started to copy my new eating behavior. He lost
twenty pounds himself.

Once you have found a Trusted Other who finds what you
are doing to be exciting and fun and agrees to help, the next
thing is to set a weight loss goal for yourself. Decide just how
much weight you do want to lose. Finally, make a contract

with yourself, either verbal or written, to lose a reasonable amount of weight in a reasonable span of time. When losing weight, especially large amounts, your best bet is to work on one pound at a time. What you do is agree to lose one pound in a reasonable, and I stress the word *reasonable,* span of time. Three to seven days falls within the limits of reasonable for many people. At the end of the allotted period, you have the option of renewing the contract or letting it lapse.

What happens if you do not lose the one pound, or maybe even gain? Nothing—you still have your option to start again. You might, though, give some thought to how attentive you were to your goal. And if you surpass your goal? *Celebrate, celebrate, celebrate!* (But not with food!)

A Trusted Other can be your confidant if you do not care to make public your goal of losing weight. You can share your secret. Keeping a secret can seem to be an awful strain at times—you just have to tell somebody! There is no need to burst when you can share.

If you and your Trusted Other are losing weight at the same time, you can provide mutual support to each other. The two of you can learn new eating habits together and compare notes on what works and what does not. There is also the possibility of two heads coming up with more ideas than one.

At this point, I would like to say a few words about groups in relation to your Trusted Other. It is possible that you do not know anyone to fill this role. Or, maybe you would like first to see how you will make out. If this is the case, you might consider joining a group weight loss program. Many people function better and accomplish more when they are supported by a group. The meetings provide everyone with a chance to sound off about what is bothering them, what is hard about staying on a weight loss program. The group and the leader become the Trusted Others.

These groups are a constant source of ideas and suggestions. Many people find them fun. Remember, though, you are the one who is losing weight, and you have to be comfortable. Where you find your Trusted Other is not important. Nor is it even essential to have one. I realize that there are many people who would not be comfortable in such a relationship. If you believe having a Trusted Other is not for you, fine. If you are not sure—well, try working with a Trusted Other and see how you like it. But should the Trusted Other concept be your thing—go to it!

8

Let's Pretend

Part of being human is having problems and being able to solve these problems in a constructive way. We come equipped with a marvelous tool that allows us to solve our problems in a creative way. I am referring to the imagination—that part of the mind that spins out ideas and images. Research seems to indicate that the two sides of the brain function in different ways. The left side is the area of automatic pilot, the things we do without conscious thought, like breathing or walking. The other side, the right side, is the creative area, the source of our thoughts and our daydreams. This right, or creative, side is the area of manual pilot.

Very few people have learned to use their imagination to its fullest potential. Of course we are constantly generating thoughts and ideas. "Would my sister like that blouse for her birthday?" "Where shall I go for vacation this year?" But what about daydreaming or fantasizing? How many people tap this natural and unique tool to create a daydream? Not all the people who could. Indeed, a lot of adults feel that imagining (creating mental pictures) is a pastime for children.

Like anything else, this attitude is learned. Society teaches that it is not adult to fantasize. Occasionally, people can get away with a little bit of daydreaming—like a young couple describing the house they hope to have. Or someone talking about the life he hopes to lead after retirement. Generally, though, most people have not learned that purposeful fantasizing is not only fun but very useful.

Many people who do use their imaginations every day go to great lengths to keep this pastime to themselves. The housewife doing a dull chore pictures herself as a famous movie star. The man mowing his lawn pictures himself as a great baseball player. Interrupt these people, and they may blush a bit and mumble vaguely, "I was thinking of something else." Never would they explain, "I was pretending I was Barbra Streisand."

Too many people have learned society's lesson so well that they never daydream; their imaginations have rusted away from lack of exercise. They may admit that they fantasized as kids, but gave up the practice when they put away their teddy bears. It is too bad, because kids have outstanding imaginations; very natural and uninhibited. Almost every little kid has an imaginary playmate at one time or another. A lot of games children play involve daydreams.

So long as it is a child who's indulging in flights of fancy, it is fine with everybody. But once the child starts to grow up and moves into the larger world, he learns daydreaming is not tolerated. In school, any kid who mentally checks out of the classroom for a few minutes is sure to be brought right back with, "Stop daydreaming and pay attention to what I'm saying!" Later on, the injunctions become even stronger. The child begins to hear statements like, "You're too old to let your mind just wander off!" or, "Only little children make up stories in their heads!" I realize that if children are to learn, they have to give attention to their teachers and studies, but they should not be completely discouraged from purposeful daydreaming. It would be far better if they were taught how and when to use their imaginations.

Fantasizing is as essential to the adult as it is to the child. In time, unfortunately, people either stop using their imaginations, or if they continue, they do so in embarrassed secrecy.

And heaven help anybody who is caught talking to himself. Again, having a conversation with yourself is a luxury only a child can afford. Talking to yourself, according to our society, is a sign of being slightly rattled.

Nonsense! Used properly, the human imagination (whether creating pictures or conversations) is an invaluable tool. Note that I said "used properly." That is what divides healthy, constructive daydreaming from purposeless fantasizing. When someone is no longer able to distinguish between reality and fantasy, there'll be a problem.

Personally, I believe we should all be encouraged to exercise our imaginations by creating mental pictures and by talking to ourselves. Talking out loud when you are alone is not as crazy as it seems. It is one way to pay attention to yourself, to acknowledge yourself, to learn the pleasure of happy talk.

"Happy talk" is a term I picked up from the musical comedy *South Pacific*. It caught my attention because I live on a Pacific island and because I like the expression. It describes perfectly what I mean. Happy talk is telling yourself nice things, making yourself feel good, pleasing yourself. And while talking out loud. Really saying the words.

It is very easy. Start out small. Practice saying your name and address out loud. Then move on to telling yourself what you are wearing. Describe, out loud, the room you are in; the furniture, the color of the walls, the rug. Then try repeating a recent conversation. The important thing is to start talking to yourself. From this small beginning, gradually expand. There is no such thing as the "right length" for these personal talks. The length is up to you. Sometimes a brief chat may suit you; at other times, a long discourse will engage your attention.

Let me explain how I use happy talk. And I do, quite often.

I might say right out, "Larry, getting into that tight parking space this morning showed a lot of driving skill. Great job!" Or, "Congratulations on that fine article you published! I'm proud of that accomplishment." I also like to relive enjoyable conversations I've had with people I care for. Quite often I repeat talks I had in Uganda, especially with my friend Sultan Karim. Happy past experiences are not gone; they can be called up whenever we like.

Another way I use happy talk is to chat with people I admire but have never met. The well-known psychologist Dr. Abraham Maslow is a man I talk to very often. I admire his work; it has played a great part in my own. So during my imaginary conversations I explain to Dr. Maslow how I am using his theories, how they worked, what modifications I've made. Things like that. It's all great fun.

Think for a moment of all the possibilities happy talk can offer. Will you feel "funny" when you start? More than likely. After all, happy talk is a new behavior, and you are not accustomed to it. Give it practice. Before long happy talk will come naturally to you.

What about creating mental pictures? With a little practice, imagery can be just as easy. As with happy talk, start out simply. Close your eyes and picture a common object. A tree, a flower, a bird. Anything. Once you have a fix on the object (let's assume you are using a tree), decide what kind of tree. How about a maple? As you get this picture in your mind, gradually begin to fill in the background.

Where is this tree? How about near a clear, bubbly stream? Are there other trees around. If so, what kind? Let's put in a few oak trees and another maple tree. What is the season? Perhaps early autumn when the leaves are turning the rich, golden shades of fall? Is anybody around? How about a group of campers? Maybe a family. What do they look like? What are they wearing? What are they doing? Pitching a tent? Just keep filling in the background. Decide how you want the details—what you want in your picture. If something displeases you, change it so you like it.

As you hold your practice sessions, you can also determine where you want to be when you are creating. Sitting down, lying down, soaking in the tub. Indoors, outdoors. And also how you want to create these pictures. Usually people find they do better with their eyes closed because the visible surroundings do not interfere with the fantasy. But not everybody does. Ron and I worked with a woman who found daydreaming more successful when her eyes were open. When she was in school, she did not want the teacher to know her thoughts were elsewhere, so she learned to daydream with her eyes open.

Do you like soothing sounds while daydreaming? Some people find that "mood" music stimulates their imaginations. Others prefer absolute quiet and find a pair of earplugs a big help. Everybody is different. It is just a matter of finding out what you like best. Experiment until you find out what pleases you the most. But how or where or when you fantasize is for you to decide. Whatever way is most comfortable for you is the right way.

What's all this fantasizing for? To help you decide on your goal. And once you decide, to help you reach your goal. For instance, to decide on your goal, it would be nice to be able to compare your options. How you look now as against how you could look. Well, you can do just that with a mental picture.

Get a picture in your mind of how some part of your body looks right now. Say your ring finger. Just visualize that finger, where the ring cuts into the flesh. Or your ankle, where the shoe strap may cut into the bulging fat. Take a good look at that image. Are you satisfied with it? Now visualize that same part of your body as it could look without the fat. That finger or ankle is thin, it is exactly the way you feel it could be. Now, in your mind, place the two images side by side. Which do you like better?

From there, visualize all of you as you are now. Take each part of your body and picture it in your mind. Put all the parts together so you see your entire body as it is at present. Next, picture your body minus all the fat. Again, take each part of your body and visualize it without the fat. Start with your toes. Picture them thin. Then go to your feet. Imagine how they will look slender. Move up to your ankles. Keep right along with each part of your body until you get to your face. After you have reviewed every feature of your body minus the flab, put all the physical parts together so you have a full-length view of the new you.

Then picture yourself in different types of clothing. You are as thin as you want to be, and you are wearing a bathing suit or form-fitting street clothes or a tennis outfit—anything you want to wear. It's like making you your own Barbie Doll. Try the new you in several outfits. The important thing is to get a firm handle on how you will look at some future date, say three months from now.

Give a great deal of attention to details. It's important to be very specific. You are not just seeing yourself thin and wearing any dress or suit. Imagine the fabric, the style, the color. Think about the shoes you are wearing. Are they loafers, high heels, sandals? What color? Are you wearing jewelry? A watch, a ring? How about perfume, cologne, or aftershave lotion? Imagine the scent. Give yourself a new hair style, a new color nail polish. Add a beard or a mustache if you want. This is the new you, and once you have lost all the unwanted weight, that is how you could look.

These "new you" daydreams can be very useful, since they can serve to clarify your goal and direction. Whenever you choose, you can turn on your favorite vision of the new you in your favorite new outfit. Then be sure to take a good, long look. Go over each detail very carefully to refresh your memory.

To be doubly sure that this daydream soon becomes reality, treat yourself to a special viewing at least twice a day.

First thing in the morning before you get out of bed, lie back comfortably and savor the vision of how you are going to look when you lose weight. Using your imagination in such a positive way even before you get up is a nice way to start your day.

Another good time to fantasize about the new you is just before going to sleep. A pleasant, positive vision of yourself will help you relax and should push any negative thoughts out of your mind. Should any thoughts of failure intrude, just notice that they are there and leave them alone. Bring out the positive. Your mind is a vast retrieval system, and you are the editor, the only editor. You bring out what pleases and helps you. The whole point of exercising your imagination is to focus on the positive, and slimming down, creating you as you want to be, is one of the most positive actions you can take.

One other way your imagination can be used to help you lose weight is by letting you enjoy the foods you want without actually having to eat them. There are going to be times while you are losing weight when you are going to want foods that you have no business eating, at least not in reality. You can, however, have these foods in a fantasy. As with the vision of the new you, you should enjoy your fantasy foods in great detail. Let's say you want an ice cream soda, or more precisely, a strawberry ice cream soda.

Start out by deciding when and where you are going to have this treat. Just after lunch? In the evening? Maybe it will be at your favorite ice cream parlor. Fine. How are you going to get there? Walk? Will you meet anybody on the way? Who? Will you talk to them? Would you rather drive? How's traffic? Any trouble finding a parking space?

Picture yourself walking into the shop and glancing around. Picture the interior in complete detail. The fountain, the booths, the clerks, even the other customers. Is it crowded? Picture what the other people are wearing. Toss in snatches of conversation. Put the vision into sharp focus.

Now take a look at yourself. How much do you weigh? What are you wearing? Fill in all the details about the star of this scenario—you! Decide where you will sit. Maybe you want to sit at the counter. Fine. Settle down and give the clerk your order. Now watch him making your soda—two scoops of strawberry ice cream, the seltzer, the cream, the flavoring, the whipped topping. Go into every detail. Right up to the cherry on top. Watch the clerk put it in front of you. Look at it for a few seconds—admire how nice and cool it seems.

Start in. Have the cherry first. Spoon it with a little whipped cream. Notice the pink streaks left on the cream by the cherry juice. Take a small sip. Imagine the cool, sweet taste. Have some ice cream. Take up the spoon and dig in. Note how the ice cream melts when you put it in your mouth. Feel it slide down your throat. Take another sip. A bit more ice cream.

Have the soda at a leisurely pace. Enjoy every drop of that ice cream soda. Savor the feeling of satisfaction as you finish it. Make the image even more real—be ethical and picture yourself paying for it and leaving the shop. Carry your fantasies right to the end. Let your imagination work for you.

Once you have finished your imaginary soda, you will find that the desire to have one in reality is gone. The craving came to you from your mind, not your body; and you have used your mind, your imagination, to satisfy that need. The beauty of eating with your mind, not your body, is that your imagination is always waiting to go to work for you. You are the producer, director, and star of the show.

Does all of this strike you as far out? It works. Believe me, it works! Michelle can testify to this, because she missed out on a fudge sundae due to imaginary eating. A few months ago, a young woman named Marcia called me one afternoon just as I was leaving my office. Michelle was waiting for me— we were going to stop off for an ice cream sundae. Oh, yes, I still eat sundaes. Only now instead of scraping the dish clean and picking at Michelle's, I leave a good deal behind.

Marcia was frantic—she wanted a chocolate cream pie desperately and had even gone so far as to call the bakery to make sure they had one in stock. Yet she did not want to give in. We talked for a bit, and then I said, "Okay, imagine you will have that pie. First decide how you are going to get to the bakery." Marcia decided to take her car, but she ran into a little traffic. There was a tie-up at one intersection. Once she got to the bakery, she found a parking space between a camper and a motorcycle. Marcia was the only customer, and she chatted with the clerk about the weather. Going into the same detail, Marcia drove home and left her car in the driveway. Once in the kitchen, she took the pie out of the box and looked at it. She especially admired the whipped cream swirls. Then she got a plate, a knife and fork, and poured herself a glass of milk. Slowly, taking up the knife, Marcia cut a piece. She described every detail to me. Then took a bite. The chocolate had a rich, dark taste and was very smooth. The cream was soft and sweet. The crust was golden yellow, light and flaky. Marcia explained every feature of that pie and how she ate it in her mind. After only three carefully described bites of pie she was too full and satisfied to continue eating.

After going through this scenario, Marcia no longer had the urge to eat the pie in reality; she had satisfied herself through imagination. In fact, she ended the conversation with, "I think I need a bicarb now." After I hung up, I looked over at Michelle and said, "Let's skip the sundae today. After hearing about that pie, I can't look at food right now." Frankly, I felt I needed a bicarb, too.

Whenever a craving appears, settle back and enjoy it. Go into details. This show is for your benefit, don't be skimpy with the scenery. Set the stage and select your supporting cast. Give them their lines, design their clothes. Pick out what you will eat. Imagine how the food will look, smell, and taste. Eat it slowly. No need to rush. By using your imagination, you can have large quantities of calorie-laden goodies several times a day and still lose weight. It is important to carry your scenario through until you have experienced the sensation of being full and satisfied; otherwise you may wish to finish it in the world of reality.

You can also use your imagination to relive happy memories—some past experience that you enjoyed, a success that made you feel good. Far too many of us dwell on our failures, things that made us feel bad. We continually call them to mind. Our imaginations are like mental television sets. It is just as easy and more enjoyable to switch on a happy program. Or to create your own pleasing mental TV shows. Super shows that make you feel like a super person.

Why not give it a try? As Abraham Maslow said, "Step out into the unknown and be creative." Create a whole new world for yourself!

9

This Thing Called Learning

Earlier on, I mentioned that the idea of learning scares a lot of people. Just say the word "learning" and a lot of people will tune out. They think learning is hard. To learn is to struggle. Whenever we are in the process of acquiring new knowledge, skills, or behavior, it does seem hard. Once we have mastered what we set out to acquire, we wonder why we ever thought it would be beyond our capacity. This is because new activities are awkward the first time around.

We tend to forget that initial period of awkwardness because, once learned, the behavior, skill, or whatever seems effortless. We come to take it for granted.

Take writing. If someone were to ask for your address, you would probably jot down the information without giving any thought to the remarkable skill you demonstrated. And without giving any thought to how awkward it was for you when you first started learning to form letters.

There is a little experiment you can do to prove my point. Pretend the hand you normally use for writing is gone. Put that hand behind your back or sit on it. Now pick up a pen or pencil with your other hand and try to write. Awkward, isn't it? Yet if you were to lose your normal writing hand, you could learn to use your other hand!

As you learn new behaviors that may help you to be thin, it will be awkward at first. You may feel ill at ease, perhaps even silly. Do not be discouraged by these initial feelings. They will disappear in a short time.

How will you go about learning thin behavior? Each of the three modes of learning—Operant, Classical, and Modeling, discussed earlier—can be used to teach yourself to be thin. But before we start discussing how to apply each mode, I want to explain first what learning is not. Usually when I begin to outline the process of learning, the person I am talking to automatically assumes what I am getting at is *unlearning* something. Nothing could be further from the truth. There is nothing to unlearn, and there are no habits to break.

I believe the whole process of learning is unidirectional—it is an add-on phenomenon. We never unlearn anything. Maybe we do not use certain skills, but we do not unlearn them. We all crawled before we walked. To learn the skill called walking, it was not necessary to unlearn the skill called crawling. The same is true when we went from riding a bicycle to driving a car. It was not necessary to unlearn cycling to learn driving. If you decided to learn another language, you would not have to unlearn English to do so.

When I was in Uganda, one of the first things that struck me about Sultan Karim was his knowledge of languages. He must have known at least a dozen, European, Asian, and African. It was fantastic. After Sultan learned his mother tongue, he just added on new languages. He never unlearned his mother tongue; he never unlearned any of the languages he already spoke to learn another. That is what learning is—you keep adding on.

It is exactly the same thing with learning to be thin—there is no need to unlearn being fat. Besides, how does one go about unlearning anyway? How can one unlearn English? You can't. And the same holds true for unlearning fat behavior—you cannot.

You *can* learn a new behavior that will allow you to leave behind the unpurposeful behavior with the other excess baggage of your past. That is what this book is all about. So now let's talk about learning a new eating behavior called thin . . .

10

Get Out Your Tape Recorder

Before you (or anybody else) can solve a problem, the problem has to be identified and isolated. Just what specifically is your problem? And what is your goal? In this case, your problem is that you are overweight. What do you want to do about the problem? Most likely your answer would be, "Lose weight." How much? Let us say, for example, seventy pounds.

With a few questions you have established your problem (overweight) as well as your goal (to lose seventy pounds). Now make an inventory of your assets, i.e., behavior that works for you. Anything that works and can help you solve your problem is an asset. Then you can make a list of your liabilities: behavior that could be a barrier to your goal. Finally, list your desired acquisitions: behavior that you have not yet learned but would like to because it may help you.

This is sort of a personal inventory; it is a big help, and it is a lot of fun to put together. Only you really know you, and only you are the expert in your problem. You have it, and you live with it. Now it is time for you to think about the problem—out loud.

You are going to sit down and make a tape recording about you. Ron and I have found that making a tape serves several useful functions. Perhaps one of the most important is that you can really listen to yourself. Often people go to a therapist and talk about their problem, which is fine, but unfortunately while talking, people do not listen to themselves. Making a tape is a way for *you* to listen closely to *you*. It will allow you to explore your problem and its development so you have a very clear picture of the issue. Then as you are solving the problem, you can refer back to the tape for encouragement and as a memory refresher. Finally, once you have solved the problem, you have a record of personal growth—you know how much you have achieved.

It is important that you use a tape recorder and not a pencil and paper (that comes later), because you want to think out loud. You want to talk to yourself in private and have a record of your conversation. And, too, most people are more comfortable talking rather than writing. Speaking words makes it easier to go into great detail. It also takes less time to say words than it does to write them.

For this project, you will need a cassette tape recorder that works perfectly. You do not want to waste time jiggling the thing, or worse, saying words that are not recorded. If you do not own a tape recorder, borrow one from a friend. If you want to avoid explanations of what you are doing, you can always say you are sending a message to a friend. Which is exactly what you are doing; you are sending a message to a good friend—yourself. You can also consider renting a tape recorder. Usually the rental fee is only a few dollars a day. You can also buy one rather inexpensively. Along with the machine, get yourself one or two sixty-minute tapes (more if you like).

Now all you have to do is block off some time to make a tape. Treat yourself to an uninterrupted hour or so and get to know yourself and your problem. If you have not used a tape recorder before, you may find it awkward. (Remember? Any new behavior is awkward at first.) Give yourself some practice beforehand, and the strangeness will disappear. The idea is to be completely natural. If you are not sure how you want to phrase something, turn the machine off and play around with the words until you find a combination you like. Plan what you will say. Use words you are comfortable with. This tape is for your ears alone, so if slang expressions are your style, use them. And forget about perfect grammar— your English teacher will never hear this. Forget, too, about trying to use professional jargon if you are unfamiliar with professional terminology.

Deal with your problem in precise terms first. *What is it?* Be as specific and as descriptive as possible. You are not just overweight, but by how many pounds? How much do you weigh? How is this a problem? Go into all the things you dislike about being fat. How long have you had the problem? What made you realize you were fat in the first place?

From your identification of your problem, go on to how you *acquired* your problem. Like anything else, you learned to be fat. How? Now how do you feel about food? Is food something you turn to when you are happy, sad, or bored? How do you feel about yourself after eating too much? Disgusted? Ashamed? Greedy? Out of control?

Okay, this is the first part of your tape. You know in your own mind what the problem is, and how it got to be a problem. Do not be surprised if you find yourself talking about things you never realized were troubling you. Chances are this is the first time you ever sat down to fully analyze the problem of your weight. Maybe you were unaware of the fact you overeat when you are bored, sad, or happy. Now that you know, this information will be extremely valuable. You can take a close look at what situations and events trigger these emotional responses. Talk about them with yourself, discuss them fully.

One woman I worked with, Sally, was surprised to realize she went on an eating binge when she was depressed. Sally knew she stuffed herself from time to time, but she never associated these binges with her depression. Once she realized the blues set her off, Sally then thought about exactly what depressed her and how she could make herself happy.

One thing that depressed her greatly was paying bills, and if she was depressed, she would eat. She then decided to flip her viewpoint of bill paying to something positive. Instead of thinking of the money she was putting out, she thought of what a good person she was for writing out those checks. With each check she wrote, Sally proved to herself and to the people she owed that her word was good. She fulfilled her promises; she met her financial responsibilities on time. A liability was changed to an asset. Her point of view was changed.

After you have discovered the types of situations that send you to the refrigerator, think how you can turn them into assets. That is what you want to do with your eating liabilities: flip them over so they become eating assets—behaviors and situations that will help you lose weight.

What emotions get you to eat? Boredom, depression, anger, frustration? How can you achieve the opposite—excitement, happiness, peace, satisfaction? Talk to yourself fully about how you can change your life so these emotions will be present. The important thing to keep in mind is that there are always answers, there are always alternatives. A heart-to-heart talk with yourself is a great way of finding them.

The next step is to *verbalize your goal*. Exactly what is it you want? Not just thin, but how thin? Do you want to lose twenty, forty, fifty pounds? Exactly what do you think will happen when you are slim? How will your life be different? Go into detail. How are you going to look once you have lost all that weight? Again, go into detail. Take yourself apart physically. Describe your face, neck, waistline, wrists, ankles—every aspect of your body without all that fat. How are you going to feel about yourself?

Now your tape is finished. Play it back several times and listen to yourself very carefully. You know what your problem is, how it got to be a problem, and what you want for yourself. The next phase does involve a pencil and paper because you are now going to make a personal assessment of your Assets, Liabilities, and Desired Acquisitions on the chart on page 69.

Assets: This column is your present. It is where you are now. You'll list here those things that work for you, that move you closer to your goal of losing weight.

The Asset column, I know, can seem difficult because we are taught that modesty is a desired social trait. Tooting your own horn is frowned upon. Consequently, we tend to push our good points into the background. We feel embarrassed about admitting our assets, even to ourselves. Worse, we convince ourselves that we do not have any. All of this is nonsense. There is nothing wrong with acknowledging our assets to anyone, least of all to ourselves. And everybody has many strong points, though they may escape notice because we take them for granted. Even if you believe you do not have any assets to use in your weight loss program, do look; you will find some! You will probably surprise yourself—you will find you have more assets than you thought.

Anything, however unimportant it may seem to you, could be an asset. Do you like lettuce? Do you dislike chocolate? Does chocolate bring out a poor complexion? Do you now drink your coffee or tea without milk and sugar? Do you like broiled meats and fish? Do you dislike fried foods? Somewhere there is an asset for you to latch on to.

Liabilities: Here is where you list the things that do not work; behavior that has not helped you achieve a weight loss. This column serves only as a reminder of the things you have already tried; think of it as a storage bin for behavior that runs counter to your goal.

Most people know what their liabilities are. Usually they spend too much time dwelling on them. There is nothing you can do about the past. What you did yesterday did not

	Liabilities	Assets	Desired Acquisitions
Thinking			
Feeling			
Doing			

Today's date: ....

My weight now: ....

My desired weight: ....

By when: ....

work—that is all. You have learned something—you have learned what not to do. Expending energy to browbeat yourself will achieve nothing.

Desired Acquisitions: This is the future column. This is where you list what you want to be and what you want to be thinking, feeling, and doing in the future. You decide how far into the future you want to project. List things that could work for you. Things that have yet to be learned. These are goals that, once achieved, could become assets.

Filling in the desired acquisitions is usually easy. We all have some idea, however vague, of what we *could* think, feel, and do in the future. Every time we say "I wish," "I want," or "I hope," we are projecting into the future. Filling in the Desired Acquisitions column should be very enjoyable.

The left-hand side of the chart is a list of behaviors. Points of view, ideas, belief systems as they relate to your own life come under the Thinking column. Your emotions are covered in the Feeling column. These are your gut reactions. In the third column, the Doing column, list how you follow through on your thoughts and feelings—what *action* you take.

Although this "game of nine" was originally developed as an inventory for sexual problem-solving, we found it just as useful for other problems. Like weight problems.

The next chart is the one I completed for my own self-evaluation. You can look it over to see just how your chart might be filled in.

After you fill in your chart, you will know what your barriers are and you can be on the alert for them. These are the attitudes that thwart you in achieving your goal. How do you rout these self-defeating attitudes? By learning new, goal-oriented behavior. Let us go back to my sample chart again and talk about the various liabilities I listed.

One of my Thinking Liabilities was believing I would hurt someone's feelings if I said no to food. That's what I believed, but I really did not know for certain, because I always took what was offered. Well, there was no rule I had to take everything. I could try a different behavior. I could handle that liability by saying "No, thank you." With few exceptions,

	Liabilities	Assets	Desired Acquisitions
T H I N K I N G	I think if I refuse food I will hurt someone's feelings. I think if I refuse food it will go to waste. I think I need a large serving of food to really get the taste. I think I have to take big bites.	I think a thin figure would be more attractive. I think people would like me more. I think I will be more acceptable.	I think I could learn to use my imagination to my own advantage.
F E E L I N G	I feel filling up on chocolate chip cookies won't matter.	I feel satisfied after a salad.	I could feel satisfied with only one meal a day.
D O I N G	I drink a lot of milk and eat a lot of ice cream.	I often skip breakfast. There are many hours in a day when I do something besides eat.	I could start liking raw vegetables like cauliflower and zucchini.

Today's date: ....

My weight now: ....

My desired weight: ....

By when: ....

people accepted my refusals. No hurt feelings, nothing. And I found another asset—saying "No, thank you" to foods that were not in line with my goal. It was the same for the other Thinking Liabilities. I no longer kidded myself. Food was not wasted because I did not eat it. And I enjoyed my food more and was just as satisfied (more so, really) with smaller servings and smaller bites.

As for my Feeling Liability—filling up on chocolate chip cookies wouldn't matter. To whom or what? Filling up on cookies most certainly did matter to my goal. They were keeping me from attaining it! So that attitude was obviously no longer tenable and a new asset, "Feeling that filling up on chocolate chip cookies does matter to my goal," was learned.

That Doing Liability was handled when I admitted that there were other things to drink besides milk. There was black coffee, tea, water. And there was always the chance to have a glass of milk in my head by using my imagination. The same was true for those ice cream snacks. There were other things, like carrot curls and zucchini strips. I went looking for alternatives that could be assets. Having found them, I then made the choice to use the positive behaviors and leave the negative ones right where they were.

The nice thing about liabilities—barriers between your goal and your present behavior—is since you put them there, you can also dissolve them. No barrier need be permanent.

How do you dissolve barriers? By really noticing your assets, using new and workable behaviors rather than old, unworkable ones, and by keeping your attention firmly on your desired acquisitions. And, most important, on your goal. Are your Thinking, Feeling, and Doing behaviors going to assist your goal? How is this done? By placing all three categories in alignment with your goal. Always ask yourself: "Is this thing I'm about to eat (or what I'm now thinking) going to help?"

As for my assets, I just went right on noticing and using them. Since I really thought a thin figure would be more attractive, the obvious corollary was: I would have to become thin. The same was true for the Feeling Assets. If a salad made me feel full, I would eat more salads. As for the Doing Assets, I went right on skipping breakfast and with no side effects. And noticing, too, that I did not have to fill my stomach to fill time. There were so many other things I could do.

The Desired Acquisitions are just that—things you want to think, feel, and do in the near future. Things that could work for you but that you have yet to learn to think, feel, and do. The Desired Acquisitions that I had listed I tried out right away. They worked and helped me reach my goal. No waiting. I did learn to use my imagination to advantage. I created mental pictures of me eating foods that were not in line with my goal. And I found I could function very well with only one meal a day. And raw vegetables turned out to be delicious. They are now among my favorite foods.

To acquire your Desired Acquisitions, just start using these behaviors. It is really that simple. When you have listed your Desired Acquisitions for your Thinking, Feeling, and Doing behaviors, just adopt them as your own—immediately.

Replay your tapes from time to time—as often as you feel you need to hear them. It will serve to keep your attention on your goal. Hearing yourself describe over and over again how you will look when you reach your goal will keep the image bright and clear in your mind.

And keep your tapes up to date. Every time you lose a few pounds, report back to yourself. Explain how you feel about your achievement. Blow your own horn long and loud. Describe how you look minus the weight you lost. Talk about how you are achieving this loss. What behaviors are you using? Are you still awkward with them or are you comfortable? Mention tactics you tried and dropped because they did not work for you, and those you have not yet learned or are in the process of learning.

As you get closer to your goal, replaying your verbal record will be a constant source of encouragement. It is also a detailed file on your personal achievement and growth. Living proof of what you can do.

Once you lose weight, what happens to your verbal records? Whatever you want to happen. You can erase the tapes, keep them, or even throw them away. I am very proud of what I did, and I think you will find that you have a feeling of self-pride and self-worth, too. And who knows, someday you may have doubts about your ability to accomplish something. If that ever happens, you can play your tapes and hear yourself talking about an achievement. My philosophy is, "If you can do one thing, you can do another." I hope in a short while that will be your philosophy, too.

11

The Operant Mode: Reward Yourself

You want to reward yourself for a behavior called "Not Eating So Much" or "Losing Weight" so you'll repeat that behavior. Rewards are necessary and desirable because they reinforce a particular behavior; if you do something that works and are rewarded, you will probably repeat it. And a reward is a good thing because you are a good person and deserve one.

All too often, fat people are very low in self-esteem. They see themselves as unattractive failures unworthy of reward or praise. They are inclined to dwell on their negative features when they should be accentuating the positive. Everybody, and I mean everybody, has good points, and they should reward and praise themselves for them. Give yourself credit, and a lot of it, for all the good qualities you possess. As you acquire even more assets, you will be able to give yourself more rewards.

One asset you want to acquire is a weight loss. To gain the reward you can exhibit a behavior that will help in your loss. Let us say you passed up dessert at lunch and dinner. That is a good, positive step toward slimming down. You could acknowledge this accomplishment with a shrug and an offhand "That's nice." Or you could really reward yourself.

We tend to be so shy about patting ourselves on the back! Bragging is viewed as a social no-no. But you can learn to acknowledge your achievements both to yourself and to others. Learn to take pride in your accomplishments, and acknowledge yourself for them at least once a day. Learning this new behavior called "Acknowledging Yourself" can help you reach your goal. Doing something positive is nothing to be ashamed of. It is just the opposite—something to be proud of. The actual reward is only important to you. Whatever pleases you at the moment is the right reward—especially if it is on target with your goal. Since you are the one who has earned the treat, you are the one who picks it.

How? There are any number of ways, and you can use one or all. Only one thing is off the reward list—foods that are not in line with your goal. The last thing you need is to fall into a pattern of forgoing a goodie at one point so you can reward yourself with it at another. Behavior like that is not moving ahead. It's standing still—it could even be moving backward. The rewards you are looking for fall into four categories:

Verbal Rewards: This is talking about your accomplishment, perhaps (though not necessarily) with your Trusted Other. There is nothing to stop you from talking to yourself about your achievement. Use your tape recorder if you like. Whatever you do, go into detail about this accomplishment. How you feel about it. Why you feel it is positive. What it has done for you. Really make use of happy talk to tell yourself how praise-worthy you are! Really listen to yourself!

Mental Rewards: Ah, the possibilities are endless. The most obvious, of course, is thinking of yourself as a good person who has accomplished something. Then there is always that marvelous built-in tool right there in your head—your imagination. Why not treat yourself to a mental vacation? Pick a place you have always wanted to visit. Settle yourself into a comfortable chair, kick off your shoes, put your feet up, close your eyes, and go! Picture yourself there surrounded by the sights, sounds, and smells of your vacationland. Bring in the people you will meet. Have conversations with them. Why not a passionate second honeymoon?

Picture you and your partner in your ideal of *the* romantic spot. After you choose the place, fill in all the details to suit your concept of the perfect setting. Candlelight, soft music, a sexy evening dress, champagne. This is your second honeymoon.

Have you always wanted a racy little sports car with four on the floor and wire wheels? Have it in your head. The whole thing—the color, the upholstery, the engine, every little detail. Then put yourself in the driver's seat and take it for a spin. Give yourself a companion to keep you company and share the thrill.

A mental reward is pulling out your favorite fantasy—one that works for you and is in line with your goal—and then enjoying it.

Physical Rewards: This could be doing something nice for yourself by doing something nice for your body. Again, there is a wide variety of possibilities—it depends on your tastes. A rubdown at a gym might be the ultimate pleasure to one person, while another would prefer a trip to the hairdresser or a manicure. Perhaps you would enjoy a nice long, relaxing bubble bath. You also have a very pleasant and powerful physical reward available to you in the form of sexual climax. During the three to seven seconds that orgasm usually lasts, you have an excellent opportunity to think of good things— how well you will look when you have slimmed down, how easy losing weight is, what you have accomplished. There you are, the new you with your love partner. Do you make a good-looking couple?

The absence of a sexual partner need not be a barrier for you. Remember: there are always alternatives. An orgasm brought about through self-stimulation can be and often is just as powerful and just as pleasurable as one brought about with a partner. If you are without a sexual partner, you can, if you wish, create one. Is there someone you think you would enjoy sex with? There is nothing to stop you from having a fantasy love affair, and using it well.

Material Rewards: You can buy yourself a present, as large or small as you like. The cost is not important—let your budget be your guide. Maybe you would rather *do* something —see a movie, call a friend, take a nap. It does not matter what it is, as long as it is something you want for yourself.

What happens if you slip off course one day? Nothing. You certainly do not want to deny or punish yourself. Doing that restricts you to a negative viewpoint. You want a positive one. So what if you slipped? A slip is something you can acknowledge with a shrug and pass by. It is not helping you achieve your goal, so don't waste your time on it.

Gradually you will come to associate your thin behavior with positive rewards. To have the rewards, you have only to stay attentive to your goal of losing weight. What nicer way to learn and practice a new eating behavior than knowing you will be rewarded with a treat?

12

The Classical Mode

The Classical Mode of learning taught me some things about food that did not prove useful for my goals: for instance, that food should be served in big portions and washed down with several glasses of milk; that no meal, except maybe breakfast, was complete without dessert. And fresh fruit was not my idea of dessert. Cakes, pies, ice cream—these were proper desserts.

Since what I had learned about food was not working, I learned new things about food that proved workable, things commensurate with my goal. I learned to eat smaller portions, to drink other beverages, to enjoy different foods. I discovered that a half dozen or so bright, fresh red cherries can be a very satisfying dessert. Oh, I know someone is going to say, "Cherries have a lot of calories. They're high in natural sugar!" I am not contradicting that point, but compared to the calories in a fistful of chocolate chip cookies or a big dish of ice cream, a few cherries are low in calories.

Through the Classical Mode you have also learned to expect consuming certain foods under certain conditions. You could just as easily have learned to expect something else under the same conditions. But you did not, you learned eating inappropriately. Now you can learn another, workable behavior—eating appropriately.

That is not as difficult as it seems. Learning a new behavior to add on to the many you already have is a matter of desire, practice, and time. Nothing says that once a behavior has been learned another cannot be learned too.

All you have to do is recognize the conditions under which you have learned to eat. The clock? Just because the time is ten in the morning or six in the evening, do you expect food? Or what about your emotions? Do you turn to food when angry, frustrated, depressed? Perhaps you associate food with certain events—going to the movies, watching a sporting event, going to a party.

Whatever sets you off, the point is that you are on automatic pilot. Under particular circumstances, you reach out for something to eat. To leave this behavior alone and begin a new one, you go to manual pilot so you can pay full attention to what you are doing. Once you have increased your ability for total awareness, you can attend to a new, workable behavior.

Let's start with emotions. Assume you reach for food when you are depressed for one reason or another. What else besides food will make you feel better? Would a friend—perhaps your Trusted Other—help? How about a long walk? Or even better, what about giving some thought to your assets? A little self-praise never hurt anybody. Negative emotions like depression, frustration, and anger come about because we put ourselves in the 0 to −10 part of the scale. Concentrating on our good points swings us over to the positive side, to emotions like happiness, pleasure, and satisfaction.

Removing depression so you will not eat is fine; putting happiness in place of a negative feeling is even better. So the next time you feel blue, instead of rushing for food, why not make yourself happy by concentrating on what a worthy person you are? Whenever you find yourself with negative feelings, rush to positive feelings instead of to the refrigerator.

Now what about time? Do you find yourself expecting food because of the clock and not because of a hunger pain? So what if it is six o'clock—who makes the decisions in your life? You or the clock? If you want a schedule in your life, there are so many other things you can do besides eat. You can watch the news on television, you can check the sports pages to find out how your favorite team is doing. The same holds true for your coffee breaks and snack times. Schedules are no reason to eat. You can learn to associate these times with another activity—like talking with your friends. The point is to be on manual pilot so you can say to yourself, "It's time for my coffee break but instead of reaching for a buttered roll, I am going to do something else. I will give this time over to keeping in touch with my friends." Then do it, and gradually coffee breaks will come to mean conversation, not food.

If you associate food with certain events, the same principles hold. Movies do not have to mean popcorn, and sporting events do not have to mean hot dogs. Instead of reaching for food, why not turn your thoughts to what a good time you are having and to the pleasure of doing something different? This way you can teach yourself to associate fun things with the pleasures of the mind instead of stomach stuffing.

The same holds true for parties. I even have an answer for the question "What else is there to do at a party but eat?" If this is how you really feel, why bother going? Would you enjoy yourself if no food was served? If your answer is no, then you owe it to yourself to find a new, enjoyable, goal-oriented behavior. Instead of eating to have fun, you could just as easily be doing something else you enjoy—an activity you do not associate with food. If your answer is yes, then you have proved that you do not need the food, so there is no need to eat it, especially if it is not in line with your goal.

Next time you have an invitation to a party, prepare yourself by picturing all the fun you will have without food. If you like, bring your own food—a nice supply of raw vegetables or fruits to nibble on. Then go and have a good time. You will probably have even more fun because you will be devoting your full energies to enjoying yourself, and not scattering them by looking for food *and* a good time.

Give thought to how you eat. Is your idea of a serving a mound of food? Would a small serving of the same food do just as well? No law says food has to be dished out with a shovel. How about dessert? Do you absolutely have to end a meal with a sweet? Does that sweet have to be pie or cake or something like that? What about fruits? Would a fruit dessert be more in line with your goal? What about dropping dessert altogether?

Am I saying these goodies must be banished from your life forever? No, certainly not! There is a way you can continue to have these foods. In your head. You can eat these foods in fantasy. You can always eat the foods you associate with certain moods and certain events in advance—in your head. What better way to satisfy yourself and not gain weight than by eating one or two hot dogs in a fantasy before you leave for the big game? Munch away until you are comfortably full in your head. Stuffing yourself, even in a mental picture, is part of your old behavior. Of course you do not have to eat mentally unless you want to. You can always go to a party or the movies, skip the food, and just enjoy yourself.

Having done all these things, remember to acknowledge yourself for your behavior. You did something wonderful, and wonderful things deserve praise—lots of it.

13

Modeling

Modeling, or learning by example, is one of the most powerful teaching aids. (Modeling is also known as vicarious, observational, or imitative learning.) Indeed, modeling is so powerful an influence that the advertising industry leans heavily on it. They hire attractive people to promote a product—men and women whom other people want to identify with and imitate.

You probably learned to be fat by watching somebody else's eating behavior. You can also learn to be thin by modeling your eating behavior after somebody else's. Somebody who is thin eats thin. Eating thin means displaying a particular behavior—a Thinking, Feeling, or Doing behavior you want to learn from someone who has successfully learned already. Modeling is very easy. You and I do it all the time.

Early Modeling: The best examples of early childhood modeling are kids who imitate their parents. The little girl who tries on her mother's clothes and spends a happy afternoon messing around with cosmetics is modeling. So is the little boy who wants to play with his father's tools. Kids who insist on having a few spoonfuls of coffee in their milk are modeling. As we grow older, we do not give up this type of learning, but our choices are broadened because we come in contact with more people.

As we reach the teen-age years, we use our peers or our heroes as role models rather than our parents. Many parents lament the way their teen-age children dress or talk. The kids' behavior merely reflects the standards learned from the peer group.

Adult Modeling: Now that you are an adult and want to lose weight, you can make a deliberate choice of a role model. You are no longer restricted by your age to parental or peer models. As an adult you have a wide assortment of people you see every day—family, friends, co-workers, acquaintances. In this group are bound to be people whose trim figures you admire; people who do not seem to have a problem staying thin. These are the people you are looking for.

Choosing Your Model: Keep in mind that it is impossible for any one person to be all things to all people. Right now, you are looking for those with an eating behavior you can use as a model for your own. Your models' other strengths and weaknesses are not important, because you are focusing on one specific behavior.

When I decided the time had come for me to lose weight, I went looking for models. At first I had no idea who could help me, but I knew who could not help me—my mother. I do not want to imply my mother is a food monster. She is not. She never never chased after me with bowls of chicken soup or anything else. She and my father did, however, believe in big servings with lots of gravy and plenty of bread to sop it up. And no meal was complete without dessert.

Well, I followed my parents' food behavior and wound up with 130 pounds I did not want or need. That does not mean my mother was without estimable qualities; far from it. Two years ago if I had decided to go into the fur business instead of losing weight, my mother would have been high on the list of possible models. When it comes to selling furs, she is one of the most successful people I know. In turn, Mom had modeled her career behavior on her father's. It is a family saying that "Marian could open a salon in the Amazon jungle and sell furs like they were dehumidifiers." Put a pelt in front of my mother, and she knows immediately if it is good, bad, or indifferent.

Selling furs, not eating thin, is my mother's strong point. That is something to keep in mind when you select your models: you want people whose strong points—in this case their eating behavior—can help you.

Actually, we usually have different models for different behaviors. For the most part my example for thin eating was Michelle, because I ate with her more often than I did with other people. There was more time to study and imitate her eating habits. For professional and personal behavior, one of my models was my good friend and colleague Ron Pion (though he soon began to imitate *my* new eating behavior— and he lost weight, too).

So while you are looking for possible models, remember: no one person will ever have all the positive traits you admire and want to acquire. Just concentrate on the qualities you would like to make your own. Remember, too, you may wish to imitate another type of behavior *after* you have lost weight. When you are thin, you may want to change the way you dress and perhaps you have observed someone who has a sense of style and fashion you want to copy. The people we use as our role models are never static; they change as we change.

What to Look For in Your Model: Essentially, you want people whose eating behavior is related to their weight. And you want a realistic relationship with them. Your favorite celebrity may have the perfect figure, but the relationship is not realistic. You may never know this successful learner personally. You may never be in a position to watch this person eat. Your model should be someone you are close to and enjoy eating with, someone you see on a fairly regular basis.

One of your models can be (but does not have to be) your

Trusted Other. In my case, Michelle helped me as both. Once I made up my mind to lose weight, I discussed my goals with her and said I wanted to watch her eating behavior and might wish to learn from her. This became a learning experience for both of us, because she had taken her eating habits for granted. Michelle was not always consciously aware of how she ate. Cutting food into tiny pieces was routine behavior for her, and she no longer thought about it. Once she became conscious of her behavior she could pay attention to mine.

Michelle is not a nagger, so she was not criticizing or picking. When she did see me gulping food, she would stop me by getting me to talk or by suggesting I take a sip of wine. Michelle was also a great source of tips. When I was learning to cut my food into small pieces, I was not sure how small small was. She suggested I cut a piece and then cut it in half.

Once you have selected people who you believe will be good models for the new eating behavior you wish to learn, you'll want to watch their eating habits carefully and copy them. You may want to tell the person you are imitating just what you're doing. If you do not know your model well enough or you think he or she will be embarrassed, spend several days watching this person eat, without being obvious about it.

Let's say your successful learner is a woman you work with, and you have lunch with her several times a week. Start out by observing what she does at coffee break. Does she reach for the pastry? If so, how many? One? Does she eat all of it? Or does she just have a cup of coffee? What does she eat at lunch? A salad? Does she leave food on her plate? Does she eat slowly? Does she pause between bites? Does she chew slowly? Once you have studied the various styles of eating thin, copy as many as you want.

Is Imitating Behavior Using People? Yes and no. Yes, because we always use other people to help us learn. As a baby you used your parents to help you learn speech. As a youngster, you learned about other things from other people. There was probably an adult you admired and said, "When I grow up, I'm going to be just like so-and-so." This is a healthy and purposeful use of other people; it is a wish to share in their particular abilities. We all do it whether we are aware of it or not.

When you select a successful learner as a role model, you are not placing any burden on him or her, you are not manipulating that person in any way. You are not exerting undue influence to make others do things they do not want to do. Selecting a model is not selfish or unethical.

Always keep in mind that by wanting to model your behavior after another person's you are really paying him or her a compliment. You're putting to use that old saying, "Imitation is the sincerest form of flattery." If you are still bothered by this concept of imitating a successful learner, remember that someone somewhere may be imitating your behavior. And once you have achieved your desired weight, someone is sure to turn to you as an example of a successful learner.

When to Choose Your Models: As soon as you decide you are going to lose weight, take an inventory of the thin people you know and have frequent contact with. Don't fall into another excuse for staying fat. You will get nowhere if you start telling yourself, "I'd like my good friend Stuart as a model, but he lives four hundred miles away, so that's that," or, "I know my golf partner, Mitchell, would be perfect, but he's away for the next three weeks." These excuses are self-defeating—and you know that!

14

Thin Foods Versus Fat Foods

I do not have to tell you about the foods that make you fat—
you know them as well as I do. You have learned to like and
eat these foods or you would not be fat. You have also
learned to associate certain foods with certain things. A coffee break means a Danish or a buttered roll. Dessert means
cake or pie—something along those lines. Snacks mean much
the same thing, and what is Valentine's Day without a box
of chocolates?

These are all fat foods. There are alternatives to fat foods
—thin foods. "Oh, here it comes," you are thinking, "he's
going to start pushing rabbit food. I hate that stuff, and besides, I'll die if I give up chocolate cake!" Well, I am not
pushing anything. The final choice is yours and yours alone.
But how do you really know you hate thin foods? Have you
ever tried to learn to like them?

You really can learn. Remember: once you had to learn
to like fat foods. And by the way, you will not die without
chocolate cake, or Danish pastry, or any other fat food. Indeed, you will not die without thin foods either, you may just
stay fat—that's all. There is no one food that is absolutely
essential to human life.

What alternatives do you have to thin foods? Fat foods and a weight problem.

For each and every place in your life you have a fat food you can learn to enjoy a thin food. Right now, today. "But I always have coffee and Danish at ten o'clock in the morning," you are thinking. Well, that's a liability. As for "always," big deal! Until you learned to read, you were *always* illiterate. That did not stop you from learning another form of communication, so why should you not learn another form of eating? What occurred in the past has nothing to do with what can occur in the future.

Let's look at thin foods and see how they bear up under close examination. Before I learned about them, I was not too interested in thin foods either. Once I took the time to study them, I discovered what they can be. Thin foods can be positively sensuous! Positively sexy! I never realized this until I sat down and took a good, hard look at a thin food.

It was a fresh raw zucchini. There was a time when I would never have eaten a zucchini. To me, zucchini was *uhgg*! Once I actually had the zucchini in my hands, the first thing that struck me was the color—a bright, foresty green. It was a natural color. All thin foods share this feature. The colors are pure and real. As I ran my fingers over the skin, I was attracted to the smoothness. Not only was it smooth; it was also cool. Then I cut into the zucchini and heard that crunch; it was crisp and fresh. The scent, as the juice trickled out, was subtle; it was there, but it was almost not there. And the taste, as I bit into the piece, was so sweet and juicy, but not sugary sweet. I was not used to the taste, so as I continued to chew slowly, I created my own experience—and did I ever! I went on chewing, slowly, really enjoying the crunchy sound and the sweet taste. Eating that fresh zucchini seemed more refreshing than drinking an ice cream soda.

Let's take a look at another thin food, maybe one that you are not familiar with. How about a giant white mushroom? Get a picture of it in your mind. It's about two inches high with a rounded cap and a short, thick stem. Look at the color first—that creamy off-white shade. It is a color that every interior decorator tries to achieve but never quite does. Such natural colors do not come from paint cans. Now, using your imagination, inhale the aroma of the mushroom. It hints of cool, green forests and pure air washed clean by a spring shower. Now what about the feel? In your mind, run your fingers over the mushroom; like white velvet—it is very soft. Turn the mushroom upside down and run your fingers over the light brown gills. This is really fun; the gills are soft and feathery. Now take a bite. Note the softness as you sink your teeth in, and the delicate flavor. The flavor is there, you know that, but you have to give it some thought. Chew slowly, savoring the thick softness of the mushroom.

Go beyond your imagination. Get yourself a few thin foods and sit down to study them. Admire the colors and the shapes. Run your fingers over them to get the feel. Inhale the scents. Chew slowly to get the full taste. Why, these are the foods that make legends. Think for a moment about a Golden Delicious apple—big, juicy, and firm. A bright, sunny yellow. This was the prize the Trojan prince Paris offered to the goddess Aphrodite. I doubt that we would have the story of Troy today if the prize had been a chocolate cake.

Studying thin foods helps you to build up excitement about them. That is part of learning to like them—being excited by a new adventure. But there is more to building excitement than feeling, seeing, and tasting new foods. There is also the buying and preparing of them. When you go out to shop for the fruits and vegetables that will help you toward your goal, make something special out of it. Make it a treat. Why not invite your Trusted Other to come along with you?

Michelle often comes with me when I go shopping for fruits and vegetables. We make a point of planning our day very carefully: the foods we are looking for, the stores we will visit. Because one of Michelle's fashion specialties is color coordination, we spend time discussing how the different foods will look next to each other. One morning not too long ago, we found a beautiful head of Manoa lettuce. This variety is grown here in Hawaii in the Manoa Valley. It's an especially delicious variety, a leafy, deep green in color with a rich, buttery taste. To enhance the particular shade of green, we looked very carefully for carrots of just the right orange tone. Giving time and thought to these small points is a terrific way to get excited about these foods. I could hardly wait to see those vegetables on a plate.

You can search out and find the best places to buy the finest thin foods. Once you find these places, take time to look over what you are buying. Select each item with care. Think of what each will do for you and how much closer it will take you toward your goal. Mix and match the different colors. Do the cucumbers look well with the carrots? Perhaps you prefer the way string beans look with carrots?

Once you have made your choices, don't just eat the food any which way. Make *preparing* the thin foods exciting too. There are so many different ways of serving a cucumber. Why not search them out and try them all? Or take carrots: they can be sliced, diced, and curled into different shapes and sizes.

How food is arranged on a plate can increase the sense of excitement, too. Even the most delicious food in the world can lose its appeal if served without thought. Take a few minutes to arrange the food on your plate. Cut the vegetables and fruits into different sizes and shapes so you can make designs. On a recent trip to San Francisco I had dinner with my good friends Stu and Davita. They served me a salad of lettuce, carrots, and cucumbers. The foods were arranged on the plate in the shape of a flower: the lettuce and cucumbers were the leaves and the stem; and the shredded carrot, the flower petals.

Granted, this was unusually elaborate, but with a little thought and help from magazines (all the big monthlies usually feature an article on serving as well as preparing foods), you can make your meals a delight to your eyes as well as to your taste buds. All of this is part of building up excitement for thin foods.

As you learn to enjoy thin foods, you may feel awkward at first, I cannot deny that. Anything new is, at first, but only because you are not used to it. So the first time you settle down to your ten o'clock coffee break and open your container of carrot curls, you will feel odd. The people around you may even comment. Don't be disturbed by this—it is normal. The first time you choose a piece of fruit for dessert instead of a piece of pastry, you will feel strange. This sense of oddness will vanish and the new behavior will become as natural as the old. It just takes a little time.

The trick with learning to enjoy thin foods is putting yourself in the right frame of mind. You always have a choice between eating a thin food and a fat food. You are hungry and want to eat, but what? Half a dozen chocolate chip cookies, or a plate of cucumber strips? Rather than dash forward to make a choice, stop and think for a minute or two. What is the fat food going to do for you? Will eating it take you closer to your goal? What is more important to you—your goal or eating the fat food? Why not eat the fat food in your mind?

Now give some thought to the thin food. Will eating the cucumber strips take you closer to your goal? How will you feel after eating them—pleased with yourself or disgusted? And the cucumber itself—how do you see this food? Visualize the fun you will have chewing slowly, separating out the seeds in your mouth. How many of those seeds can you split with your teeth? Why not make a bet with yourself on the number you will be able to split?

Most people are turned off by thin foods because of their point of view. Once the view is switched over from "rabbit food" to sensuous thrill, the sense of anticipation and excitement follows naturally.

Does this mean you will never be able to eat your favorite foods again? I cannot really answer that question, but I doubt very much that you will have to banish all goodies from your life. As you move along toward your goal, you will find foods that work for you. You may find you can have a slice of pizza occasionally. You will also find, though, that there are fat favorites that just do not work for you. To achieve your goal, you will have to drop these foods from your eating pattern. A food that gets in the way of your goal is a drag; why would you want to be saddled with it?

I firmly believe that if you treat yourself to the adventure of learning to eat thin foods, you will have more fun than you ever did with fat foods. Why not give yourself permission to try? You have nothing to lose but your fat! I did it, and it worked for me!

15

Eating Thin

Thin people are different from fat people. That does not sound like a very brilliant statement. Anybody with eyes can see that the thin weigh less. They do, certainly. That is the most obvious difference; but there are other differences too. Thin people feel differently about food, very differently; and more important, they eat differently. If that sounds weird to you, you can check it out for yourself.

Find someone you consider slim and watch him or her eat—really watch. Most people who do not have a weight problem take their time finishing a meal. They usually eat slowly, taking small bites. There is none of the gulping food that fat people indulge in. Slender people really taste their food; they enjoy it. Usually, heavy people do not. That is because thin people chew, and I mean chew, their food.

I can remember back in the days when I was fat how quickly I ate. I was always the first one finished. I would be plowing through a second helping before the other people at the table had finished their first serving. And I never really tasted anything. It was strictly shovel the food in and swallow it down. In and down.

Stopping when I was full was not my style in those days either. Once Michelle, our friends Stu and Davita, and I went

94

to a popular Honolulu restaurant for dinner and I stuffed myself to the point where I had no room for dessert. Rather than pass up dessert, I left the table and walked in the restaurant garden for fifteen or twenty minutes. When I felt I could eat more without bursting, I returned to the table. No way was I going to leave the restaurant without dessert!

When I started seeing Michelle, I remember being struck by how long it took her to finish her dinner. And it was not because Michelle was doing all the talking, either. I was doing most of the talking and nearly all of the eating too. It was by watching Michelle eat that I learned how thin people eat. At first I thought she took those tiny bites because she was used to eating with chopsticks, but as I looked around it became obvious that most slender people take small bites of food.

Michelle is also a thorough chewer. I was not, but without chewing slowly and carefully you will never really taste the food you eat. And unless you really taste your food, you will never know if you like it. Since our taste buds are located on our tongues, the food has to be in the mouth for a while. The gulp-and-gobble style of eating pushes food right past the taste buds. Consequently, the full flavor of food is often missed.

Learning if you really like what you eat is important in losing weight. When I was heavy, you may remember, I had a thing about chocolate chip cookies. A dozen at a sitting was not unusual for me. Even when I started with the notion of having just one, somehow it always became ten or twelve. Then I started chewing thoroughly to get the full taste. At that point, I discovered that I did not really care for chocolate chip cookies as much as I thought I did. When they were fresh, they were too soft; and when they were stale, they were too dry. Once you start savoring your food to get the full taste of each bite, you will be amazed at the number of things you discover about flavor and texture. I still like chocolate chip cookies. I still eat them, but with an increased awareness. I can discriminate between one and twelve because my eating behavior is on manual pilot.

Another thing I noticed about Michelle (and thin people in general) is that they pause between bites. The knife and fork are put down on the plate. When I first started watching closely as she ate, I noticed Michelle had a ritual that I thought came from her Japanese culture. After chewing a piece of food, she puts down her knife and fork. Then she joins in the conversation. Fat people, since they are so busy stuffing themselves with food, or worse, planning to get more, do not take time to enjoy table talk.

That's how I was. While eating, very rarely did I pay much attention to what the others at the table were saying. I missed a lot of good conversation when I was heavy. Meals can be so much more enjoyable and relaxing when you share words as well as food with others. When fatties eat, they are stingy with words as well as greedy with food. If they do talk, others often have trouble understanding them because they talk with their mouths full.

After she has contributed to the conversation, Michelle has a sip or two of whatever beverage is served with the meal. Unlike fat people, thin people are very leisurely about getting back to their food. And why not? The food is not going anywhere; nobody is going to snatch it away (unless you are eating with a dedicated fatty).

Then Michelle has a few more sentences to add, and I mean sentences. Before I started copying her eating style, my table talk consisted of a few grunts, "Oh, sure," "uhmm," "yeah," and "I guess." Listen to yourself, really listen, the next time you eat. Probably you are doing the same thing. How would you like to be chatting with someone who is giving only half an ear, if that, to what you are saying? It's not very pleasant.

Once this cycle has been completed, then and only then does Michelle take another bite of food. She acquired her eating habits the same way you and I acquired ours—by imitating her parents and her brothers and sisters. Her whole family eats the same way, and the whole family is thin.

This leisurely manner of eating has another advantage—it is far more attractive than the way fat people eat. I never realized how unattractive my former eating behavior was until I saw myself in a mirror. I had been watching not only thin people eat, but also fat people. I wondered how my eating style looked to others. So I put a mirror on the table and watched myself. It was quite an eye-opener. I was pushing large pieces of food into my mouth. And at a good pace. I could see quite plainly that I was not enjoying the food—I was too busy wolfing it.

Buy a mirror and put it in front of you the next time you eat. I think you'll be equally taken aback at your reflection.

Another important facet of eating thin to be thin is: do one thing at a time. Don't eat and read, or do a crossword puzzle, or watch television, or talk on the telephone. By trying to do two things at the same time, you do an injustice to yourself. Are you using your energies to enjoy your meal —or your book or TV program or whatever? If you are truly attending to what you are eating, then what you are reading or watching is neglected. If the reverse is true, then how can you enjoy and savor your food?

Eating can be a pleasure just as reading, working out puzzles, watching television, or chatting with friends can be a pleasure. To get the most from them, you have to give your full attention to them, one at a time. There is no sense trying to do more than one thing at a time; you are only cheating yourself of enjoyment.

Of course, new eating habits are not learned immediately. The first few times you feel awkward. Remember when you were learning to drive a car? You just couldn't get your foot to give the engine the right amount of gas. Either you pushed the accelerator down too far or not far enough. And the first time you stepped on the brake pedal, you and your instructor nearly went through the windshield.

Learning a new eating pattern also takes a little bit of getting used to. With minimal practice and a high degree of excitement, your newly learned eating behavior can soon be as natural as the old one. After all, today you hop in your car and drive away without flooding or stalling the engine. You brake to a stop smoothly. There is no awkwardness. As with most things we do well, we hardly ever notice how well we do them. A thin eating style will be like that. Once you have mastered it, you will be hard pressed to remember when eating thin was awkward for you.

"Ahhh," you might be thinking, "all this chewing, taking small bites is fine, but the talk breaks are out because I live alone." Living alone does not have to be a barrier to thin eating at all. In fact, it is a great way to exercise your imagination, because you can talk to yourself in the privacy of your own home. You have happy talk to use.

Yes, mealtime is a perfect time to treat yourself to a session of happy talk. Tell yourself about your assets, especially all the new ones you have acquired. Give yourself an imaginary dining companion if you like, perhaps a close friend or relative you haven't seen in a while. Talk over past joys. Review your cherished memories.

You could also pretend you are eating with someone you admire and would like to meet. Say the things you would if you met this person in reality. Who knows, maybe you will someday.

Or you can tell yourself about the wonderful vacation you have planned. All the sights to see and the people to meet. If you have just returned from vacation, tell yourself all about it. Where you went, who and what you saw, what you did.

Doing something like this when you eat alone serves a dual purpose. It slows down your eating, and it allows you to clarify your thoughts by verbalizing them. And it gives you more practice with using imagery and happy talk. Make up talking games if you wish. Be creative. Remember, the game is yours. You make the rules. Use the tool of your imagination to create the games you like. Part of the fun comes from deciding how you will use your capacity for fantasy to slow down your eating.

The next question is: Where are you going to be doing your thin eating?

Just as there is a fat eating style and a thin eating style, there are fat eating places and thin eating places. Fat people eat anywhere and everywhere. I have even heard of one man (not me!) who would have two cans of beer and a big bag of potato chips while soaking in the tub.

Before I lost weight, I ate wherever there was food. I did not walk through a shopping center without stopping at at least three snack bars. The glove compartment of my car was stocked with handy bags of peanuts and candy bars. It did not matter whether I was standing up, sitting down, walking —if there was food around, I ate it. If there had been a way to pull it off, I probably would have eaten while I was sleeping.

Thin people usually do not eat this way at all. They usually eat at one place and one place only. At a table that is set with a knife, fork, and spoon. They rarely eat while window shopping or standing in the kitchen cooking or lounging in bed. This is like the classical learning we talked about earlier. The dog began to salivate when he heard the bell. For thin people, a place setting at a table means "It's time to eat." Any other situation does not trigger an eating response.

Once you have learned to eat only at a table while sitting down, you will probably not want to eat any other way, especially if this behavior is assisting you with your goal. To do this, it is a matter of asking yourself if that stand-up snack bar is a good place to eat consistent with your goal. And the likelihood of losing weight is no. Once you have learned to associate eating with sitting down at a table, you will not want to eat any other way.

To further slow down your eating speed, you may find it useful to eat with your other hand. If you are right-handed, hold the fork in your left hand. A number of people have told me that using chopsticks is a great help. It also allows you to learn a new and very fashionable skill.

These suggestions may seem odd to you. I make them only because they have worked, not only for me but for others. A number of people who have lost weight say how helpful the techniques of thin eating proved. But remember: the new and different often require a turnabout in viewpoint before they can be appreciated. You are used to seeing food and eating it from one perspective; now another is offered, and this is a radically different perspective from the one you are familiar with.

However odd these suggestions may seem to you, they will never become familiar and comfortable unless you put them into use. Just reading about them will not move you one step closer to being the thin person you want and deserve to be.

16

A Sense of Timelessness and a Feeling of Selfulness

What happens if you decide you are going to lose fifty pounds in six months and the six months pass and you have not lost the entire amount? Maybe you have lost only forty pounds or only twenty-five. Does this mean you are a failure, that you won't reach your goal? Does this mean you should forget the idea of slimming down? Does it mean anything at all?

Yes, it does have meaning. It means you should not get yourself too wrapped up in the question of time, especially if you are moving toward your goal.

Time is an artificial measurement created to serve us, not for us to serve it. Time is merely a convenience that allows us to order our lives. Somewhere along the way, mathematicians decided that we needed time (and we do), so they divided a year into 365 days with each day of twenty-four hours and each hour of sixty minutes. People measure time in different ways. In some societies a day is measured from sunrise to sunrise; in others from sunset to sunset; in ours from midnight to midnight. It's all arbitrary, and, to be sure, useful.

A day could just as easily be thirty-six or even forty-eight hours. A month could be sixty days instead of thirty. These arbitrary units exist only to give form and order to our lives. If you are catching an 8:22 A.M. plane and you know you live about an hour's drive from the airport, these artificial divisions enable you to plan so that you can make that flight. A way of measuring is necessary and useful for many facets of our lives. I said "many," not "all." During a weight loss program, you want to acquire just the opposite of a sense of time—you want a sense of timelessness.

This means you are not a slave of time. The amount of time it takes for you to lose weight is not important. However long it takes, it will not be soon enough. Most everyone I know, myself included, wants or wanted to be thin yesterday. Nobody wants to wait for the future. The future is too far away, especially if the past is filled with failure. Six months seems like an eternity, and after investing all those weeks, you want results! Okay, let us discuss some ground rules about timelessness, primarily what it is and how it is achieved.

1. *The more weight you want to lose, probably the longer it will take.* This seems straightforward enough, but you would be surprised at the number of people I meet who announce they want to lose fifty pounds in three weeks. It may have taken three years to put on that excess weight, but that does not matter. Well, you know that it will take a while to lose weight. As you move along and lose weight, at whatever rate, use your imagination well and acknowledge what you are doing and have done.

2. *Do not compare yourself with another.* Maybe your Aunt Ethel lost twenty pounds in two months. If she did, that's terrific. But just because she did does not mean you will, or that you have to. Perhaps you will discover that in eight weeks you have lost fifteen or thirty pounds. You will reach your goal soon enough. The important thing is for you to lose weight without holding yourself to somebody else's routine.

3. *Do not dwell on an artificial deadline.* Rather than saying "I must lose fifty pounds in six months," set your immediate goal in small steps like "I am going to lose fifty pounds, and I am going to do it one pound at a time. My goal is one pound a week." That's it. Period. Don't use time as a

hard-and-fast guide. When you restrict yourself to a specific amount of time, you are building a barrier to your own success. If fifty pounds in six months is your goal, what happens if you do not meet it? Do you forget about the reducing program? There is a good chance you will. Your purpose, remember, is to lose weight, not to beat the clock.

4. *Use time as a benchmark of progress.* Suppose six months have passed. You wanted to lose fifty pounds, but you step on the scale and find you have lost only thirty-five. Is this failure? No way! Look at what you have achieved. Accentuate your achievement, acknowledge what you have accomplished. In six months you have become lighter; you moved forward. Something was accomplished through your efforts. If you have moved toward your goal in six months, another month will bring you even closer. Each day you adhere to your purpose, you move that much closer to your goal.

5. *Always remember: the future will arrive before you know it.* Often when someone tells me, "I want to lose fifty pounds. How long will it take?" my only answer can be, "As long as it does." This honest answer can bring forth a shocked "What does that mean?" It means just that. I realize the future always seems a long way off, until it arrives. When an attitude like "It will take too long" presents itself, I then ask the person to think back maybe six or seven months to what he or she was doing. An answer like "I was on vacation then—that seems like only yesterday" is common. I can then mention that if the weight loss program had been started then, probably the goal would have been reached by now. That six months in the future will be here before you know it.

I also ask, "What else do you have to do with your time but lose weight?" If all our problems were solved yesterday, we would have nothing to do with ourselves. It's not uncommon for people to keep problems around just to have something to talk about. There are even people who deliberately create problems to have something to do or to solve. People do things at different speeds. Rather than let yourself get bogged down in how far away the future is, turn your attention to how quickly time can pass. This is using your past in a constructive way; you know from previous experience that time flies, therefore you can assume it will continue to do so. You will be thin before you know it.

6. *Achieving your goal, and not the amount of time it takes to achieve it, is the important thing.* Direct your attention and energies to losing weight. A weight loss is a weight loss whether you achieve it in three months or in six months.

7. *Make time your servant.* Rather than saying "I must lose fifty pounds in six months," break time down into small, manageable units. Set a series of subgoals based on weeks. Be realistic: one pound in, say, three to seven days. Plan to drop one pound at a time. At the end of the time span, evaluate your loss. If you exceeded your goal, terrific. Decide if you want to try to equal or exceed it the following week. That is your choice.

Even if you fall short of your goal, accept whatever you did lose for what it is—an accomplishment—and evaluate your goal once again for the next week. You might want to try dropping your weekly goal to half a pound or a quarter of a pound. You might want to have your subgoal remain the same and evaluate your food intake instead. Review the week and decide if you were attending to your goal as carefully as you might.

That is how to produce a feeling of timelessness. You cease to dwell on time, and therefore time does not become a barrier. Your purpose is to slim down, and this is where you concentrate your energies. The time it takes to achieve your goal is not important at all. The funny thing is, the less thought you give to the amount of time involved in losing weight, the faster you will probably shed those unwanted pounds.

Along with a sense of timelessness, you want to achieve a

feeling of *selfulness*. Many people, and not all of them fat either, have a difficult time praising themselves. We all know our liabilities and faults, but ask someone about their strong points or their assets and nine out of ten people will not be able to answer without hesitating. We learn this because our upbringing stresses modesty. People who go around talking about the things they do well are usually dismissed as conceited, self-centered, egotistical. How many people do you know who say "I'm a super mechanic," or "I'm an excellent secretary," even if the statements are true? More than likely you hear things like "I don't know as much as I should about diesel engines," or "I'm lousy at filing."

All too often we downgrade or (worse) ignore our talents and draw attention to our faults and weaknesses. Fat people are very likely to do this. They lock themselves into the negative side of their lives. This is the 0 to −10 side of the scale. There they stay. They think of themselves in terms of "I'm just a fat slob," or "I feel like a pig every time I eat," or "I'm ugly to look at." And they often act as if these statements *are* true.

How do you feel about yourself? Do you feel negative? Do you think, feel, and act as though you are without assets of any kind? If you do, it is probably time to switch your point of view as well as your feelings and actions from the negative to the positive. People whose outlook is consistently negative are restricting their lives; they are also missing out on the joys of what I call selfulness—being full of yourself, full of your assets.

This being full of yourself is a feeling of self-appreciation, the act of praising your good points, thinking about your good features. It is liking yourself and becoming even more likable in your own eyes. How is this done? One way is by setting up little challenges for yourself to prove you can achieve things—positive, good things.

First you have to acknowledge your present assets—what

you do really well already. If you're thinking, "That's impossible. There isn't one thing I do well," you are very wrong! We all have something we're good at.

If you are having trouble *finding* your assets, go back to basics, as we did before. It is so easy not to notice the things we do well because we take our abilities for granted. What about your home—are you a super housekeeper? Or your job—do you have it because of some special skill? Are you good at crossword puzzles or anagrams? Maybe you play the meanest game of gin rummy on your block. Are you always elected treasurer of your club because you are the only member who understands the mysteries of a bank statement? If you poke around long enough, you will find an asset—or two or three, or many, many more.

Once you find your assets, you have your foundation. Now you can begin to work up small challenges for yourself and acquire even more strong points. You are ready for the "game of nine." This game is based on the chart shown on page 107. It is the same one used in Chapter 10.

To play the game, you do essentially what you did with the first chart. List your liabilities. Put them down on paper and leave them there. Now list your assets—any assets; if they are of a kind that will help you reach your weight goal, that's even better. The last thing is to list the things you want in the near future—these are your desired acquisitions, the things you could learn to think, feel, and do, but haven't yet. The game consists of moving the Desired Acquisitions column into the Assets column. You can also move your Thinking, Feeling, and Doing behaviors up and down the chart. You can take a Doing behavior and make it a Thinking behavior by using your imagination. Two completed charts are given on page 108. They were filled in two weeks apart. Quite a difference in just fourteen days!

The purpose of the game is to concentrate on your Thinking, Feeling, and Doing assets so you can acquire what you want. The woman who filled in the two charts had a lia-

	Liabilities	Assets	Desired Acquisitions
Thinking			
Feeling			
Doing			

bility: she felt antisocial when she refused food. Her asset: feeling excited about being thin. To feel proud about a five-pound weight loss, she had only to leave her liabilities alone. That's right, she didn't have to do anything with them. She used her sense of excitement, not her liabilities. She had a choice. She could have used either behavior. There is no choice until both behaviors are learned.

Once you obtain the Desired Acquisitions, they become Assets. You shift them into the Assets column. When all three Desired Acquisitions become Assets, you have won the game, and you can start again. By playing the game of nine, you are constantly building up your assets and electing not to use

FIRST CHART

	Liabilities	Assets	Desired Acquisitions
Thinking	I think I need bacon every time I have eggs.	I think I can lose weight.	I think I could be better-looking thin.
Feeling	I feel antisocial if I refuse food at a party.	I feel excited about losing weight.	I could feel proud of myself if I lost 5 pounds and could fit into a smaller size.
Doing	I eat too much candy to lose weight.	I do eat cauliflower.	If I want candy I could eat it in my head so as to eat less in reality.

SECOND CHART

	Liabilities	Assets	Desired Acquisitions
Thinking	I think I have to use butter.	I think I can lose weight. I think I can lose even more weight.	I could learn to think butter is unnecessary.
Feeling	I feel food tastes better with a lot of butter.	I feel excited about my 5-pound weight loss.	I could feel good about myself if I use less butter.
Doing	I do use too much butter.	I do eat cauliflower. I am eating less candy.	I could learn to use less butter.

your liabilities. You are proving what a worthy person you are. Each game you win increases your worth because you will be choosing more assets and fewer liabilities. You can call on your old behavior any time you want, but you will probably find that you are not using your old behavior patterns because they are not in line with your goals.

When you turn your full attention to your strong, positive features and actively seek more, you are filling yourself up with the good you—you are becoming full of self. In effect, you are saying to yourself, "Yes, I have liabilities, but I prefer to choose my assets. They do more for me. They are more in line with my goals."

Concentrating on your liabilities achieves nothing toward realizing your goals. Concentrating on your assets can achieve everything.

17

A Myth Is As Good As a Smile

I admit to a fondness for myths and legends; when I was a kid they made up some of my favorite bedtime stories. The trouble with myths and legends, though, is that sometimes they cross over from the world of fantasy to the world of reality.

Sometimes believing a myth does not cause difficulty. Who knows? Maybe there really is a Santa Claus living with eight reindeer at the North Pole. Anyone who has noticed the excitement of kids during the holidays realizes that myths can bring happiness.

Unfortunately, myths about weight loss can do a lot of harm if taken seriously, because they become barriers to achieving the weight you want. Truth, generally, is our point of view. If the viewpoint is that baked potatoes are tasteless without sour cream, that can become "truth"—and a barrier. The point of view, and therefore truth, could just as easily be: baked potatoes need nothing added to taste delicious.

The myths I discuss here are not the only ones in circulation. They're just some of the more popular ones. It would take a whole book to cover every misconception about weight loss. The central theme running through almost all of these popular beliefs is that you have no control over how much you weigh. It's hoped that as you read on, the last remaining barriers standing between you as you are now and the slim body you want and deserve will fall away.

1. *If a food tastes good, it's high in calories.* This all-encompassing statement means nothing because it does not define what "good" is. What tastes good is a very personal thing. Chocolate cake is high in calories, but there are people who hate the taste of chocolate and never eat it. Cucumbers are very low in calories, yet there are people who swear cucumbers are the most delicious food in the world. The trouble with this myth is that some people believe they must eat foods they dislike; they believe this is the way to shed pounds. Sour cream is a perfect example. Thousands of people use sour cream even though they can't stand the stuff. If they hate it, therefore it must be low in calories. No way! A serving of sour cream has exactly the same number of calories as an equal serving of sweet cream. People also stuff themselves with liver even though they detest the taste. Liver *is* a low-calorie food, but it is not the only one. Chicken, turkey, veal, and tuna fish are too, especially if you leave off mayonnaise and heavy sauces.

The last thing you want to do is stop eating foods you like. You could cut down on these foods. Even better, have these foods in a fantasy (eat in your head, not in your stomach). There is also the opportunity to be creative about food. Investigate new ways of eating. I was once convinced every vegetable needed butter. Then I tried eating them without butter, and discovered a new taste treat. Today I prefer to enjoy the full flavor of vegetables. From my present point of view, butter only masks the flavor.

2. *Fat people are neurotic.* I suspect this blanket statement was worked up by a parlor psychologist who had a murky knowledge of human behavior. Just what is "neurotic" anyway? It is a label that is of no assistance to either fat or skinny people. If we must use labels, let's make them of assistance to people! The reasoning behind this useless statement is that

fat people are in an emotional mess because they cannot control their eating. They will never be thin until they find out why their emotions are in a turmoil. This becomes a barrier to being thin because people can say, "I can't afford long-term analysis to find out what my problem is," or "I don't have the time to give." The problem of being overweight has nothing to do with a neurosis; it has nothing to do with whether or not you're afraid of spiders. It has to do with using a learned eating behavior that promotes overweight. Once you learn a new repertoire—thin eating behavior—the weight problem can soon disappear.

3. *A woman is going to gain weight each time she has a baby.* Only if she allows it to happen. No law of nature ordains that a woman has to gain several pounds every time she has a baby. Like other myths, this is a barrier to slimness. If a woman stays on manual pilot during and after pregnancy, she need not gain weight. Woman who are not physically ill but gain excessive amounts of weight during pregnancy are often those who believe in "eating for two." While I am on the subject, I will say a few words about this myth of "eating for two." It has a similar learning history as the excuse I used to spout, "I need all that food so I won't pass out in the operating room." The myth sounds good and seems hard to challenge. But just as I would rationalize eating a box of cookies with "I can't risk fainting," many pregnant women justify an extra helping of mashed potatoes or a second dessert with "Half for the baby and half for me." This will not wash—eating for two is another excuse for eating too much. The same thing goes for cravings. These are learned behavior. We hear so much about odd cravings for ice cream at three in the morning that we expect them. And what we expect tends to happen. Should you crave ice cream, why not satisfy it with a fantasy?

4. *While reducing, it's best to weigh yourself once a week.* Weigh yourself every day, and not just once. Two, three, or even twenty times a day! When I was reducing I weighed my-

self on every scale in the hospital at least once a day. Every time I passed one, I would hop on. I weighed in wearing a scrub suit, wearing street clothes, wearing shoes, barefooted. A scale is the only source of biofeedback you have, and you cannot get the information unless you step on the scale. But, wow! The excuses for not getting on that scale! I have been told, "I don't own a scale," "My scale doesn't work right," "My bathroom is small. I don't have room for a scale." Sorry, but a bathroom scale can be bought at a fairly low price in almost any corner drugstore. And no law says you have to keep a scale in the bathroom. What's wrong with the kitchen? Or right next to your bed?

Another excuse I hear often is, "I can't read the dial because my stomach gets in the way." If this is your reason for not stepping on a scale, I can only ask, "There is not one single person available who can read the dial for you?" I have also been told, "If I weigh myself a lot, I won't see any prog- ress, and I'll get discouraged." There is no excuse for not knowing. Some people can tell more accurately how much gas they have in their cars than how much weight they have on their bodies. It's better to know what is happening with your body. At least you know you're not gaining weight. You will know what you weigh, and you can interpret this information.

For example, some women gain a pound or two just prior to menstruation. How is a woman to know if a slight weight increase is due to a normal physical cycle or lack of attention to her goal unless she plots this monthly gain? By hopping on the scale many times a day, she can determine any slight gain or loss and stay on purpose. If she sees a small increase in weight every twenty-eight days, she knows hormone shifts, and not overeating, might be causing a case of temporary water retention. But suppose you indulge in a heavy Italian meal one evening and step on the scale the next morning and see a quarter-pound that was not there the day before? Im- mediately you will know Italian food is not helping you reach your goal. Besides, I feel it is far better to find a quarter-pound gain right away than to wait seven or ten days and find an extra few pounds.

Several daily trips to the scale will allow you to spot problems before they become more troublesome. When you weigh yourself infrequently, you run the risk of drifting away from your goal without realizing it. Another popular excuse is "It's too much trouble to weigh myself." Nonsense! Stepping on a scale is less trouble than going to the toilet. So do get on the scale, and often. Small increments of weight loss can make you feel proud of your achievements and assist you in staying "high" during your day.

5. *Everybody gains weight as they grow older.* Oh sure, just like sex ain't as good as it used to be. I lost weight as I grew older. Gaining weight is most definitely not part of aging, although it certainly can occur that way.

How come so many people put on pounds as they grow older? Primarily because they become less attentive to what they eat. Housewives may fall into the rut of the afternoon coffee klatsch which often features cookies and cake; the middle-aged man parks himself in front of the television set with a few cans of beer and a healthy serving of peanuts every evening. After a while, these careless eating habits show results in the form of a spare tire around the waistline or what is called middle-age spread. Your eating behavior, not your age, is the cause of a weight gain.

6. *Some nationalities are predisposed to fat.* Your ethnic heritage does not guarantee that you will be fat or slim, but it's sad to see how many people believe this. Several months ago, while I was out to dinner with friends, the conversation got around to weight, and a young woman in our party expressed concern about her figure. Since she did not show signs of a weight problem, I suggested she keep eating as she was because her present eating behavior was obviously working. "Oh, no, Larry," she said, "no matter what I do, I'll be fat in ten years. I'm Italian, and Italian women always get

fat." This woman was the victim of a myth and truly believed she was doomed to a fat future because of her ancestry. She was firmly convinced that if she was of Danish extraction, or anything else but Italian, she would have nothing to worry about. Your ancestry or your genetic make-up have nothing to do with your weight.

What can make you fat is your cultural background, but that is very different. Some cultural groups admire fat people. Lots of padding is thought to be a sign of health, wealth, or both. The old Hawaiian culture regarded huge amounts of weight as a sign of power. You have no control over your genetic heritage—the color of your hair, the shape of your eyes, are a matter of chance. Your cultural heritage is something you can control because you acquired it after you were born. If you learned one life style, you can learn another. If you were raised in a cultural background that stressed large quantities of fat food, you can just as easily learn another pattern that stresses thin foods.

7. *You will gain weight if you stop smoking.* I used to believe this myth myself. Then I decided to test it. While I was reducing, I stopped smoking and went right on losing weight. You see, many people who stop smoking substitute eating for smoking. When people stop smoking and start showing a weight gain, it may be because they are looking for something to do with their time. No longer able to reach for a cigarette for gratification, they reach for food instead. They haven't learned to choose a nonsmoking behavior. Giving up smoking does not mean an automatic weight gain. The fact that you stopped smoking has nothing to do with your weight. What and how you eat does.

8. *Your job has a lot to do with what you weigh.* That is a nice comforting myth. "I sit at a desk all day. That makes me fat, not what I eat." If this were true, how come everybody who works at a desk is not fat? If working at a desk makes people gain weight, people who earn their living doing physical labor should all be thin. Right? Wrong. Next time you

walk by a construction site, take a good look. I can almost guarantee you will see men working there who are overweight. Whether you work at a desk or haul steel girders for a living, you will gain weight only if you eat too much. To reduce, you do not have to change your job; you only have to alter your eating behavior.

9. *Hot food is better than cold food.* I don't know in what way hot food is better. Nobody ever told me about any magical properties in hot food. I do know that people who believe this tend to eat faster. Therefore they eat more than people who do not. Because of the rush to eat the food while it is hot, the meal is shoveled down. Without slow, deliberate chewing and swallowing, a full feeling does not come as quickly. Therefore you eat more. Give your food a chance to cool off; eat slowly. (And you'll be less likely to burn your tongue!)

10. *Losing the first ten pounds is always the easiest.* Supposedly the first ten pounds or so are water loss. Water loss goes quickly—or so it is believed. Don't let this myth steal the credit. Those first ten pounds or so were lost *because you made them disappear.* Your efforts alone were responsible. Those first pounds seemed to go quickly because you were not yet bored. Sure, all the little gimmicks of weight loss seem like fun when new, but after several weeks eight glasses of water or four grapefruits a day can be pretty dull. So losing seems hard because boredom sets in. I firmly believe if a consistent level of excitement is maintained, all the pounds will seem easy to lose.

11. *We need plenty of milk.* For what, I now wonder. Before I lost weight, I went through at least two quarts a day. Now I rarely drink milk. And I'm getting along just fine. No brittle bones, no loose teeth. Yet some people faithfully drink milk every day believing they are doing themselves a favor. Even people who cannot stand milk force it down. Sometimes they lace the milk with calorie-rich flavorings. They would be better off if they stopped forcing themselves to

drink something they hate. No food is absolutely essential to human well-being, and that includes milk.

12. *Less food will make you dizzy and weak*. For years I told myself I needed every crumb I shoved down my throat. If I did not eat a lot of food, I would get dizzy and faint. I had no proof; I just assumed it would happen. The chances are very good you will not pass out from hunger unless you continually tell yourself that you will. Oh, yes, you can talk yourself into feeling faint. The only likely result if you eat less is that you will lose weight. Generally, we consume much more food than we really need to survive. Overeating becomes the norm, and we come to believe that anything less than the norm (which is too much in the first place) will cause problems. Before long, a vague notion is accepted as fact even though it has never been tested for validity.

13. *I was caught off guard*. This is another one I hear very often, and I used this myth a lot, too. Usually the explanation is, "I was caught off guard because we went out to eat." I can understand this; I was always being caught off guard myself. I would be checking a new mother in the maternity ward who would say to me, "Would you like a chocolate-covered macadamia nut?" It never occurred to me to say, "No, thank you." Now when I hear this myth, I ask, "How were you caught off guard?" The answer is usually something like, "Well, what else could I do in a restaurant but order a big meal?" This will not wash. The whole idea of a restaurant is choice. A menu offers a wide selection of food—some will fit with your goals and aspirations and some will not.

You have to make a choice. Do you want a meal that will move you closer to your goal or one that can hinder you? Nobody is caught off guard where food is concerned. You will not be asked to leave any restaurant because you order a light meal; you will not break the law if you refuse food or leave some on your plate, rather than in your gut. Deep down inside you know this, too. When you let yourself be duped by this myth, you are setting yourself up, as I was, as a food patsy. Why should you set yourself up as a patsy for every bit of food around? Always keep in mind that there is a choice, and it is yours to make, once you learn a new behavior.

14. *I have to feed my stomach disorder*. This myth is a current favorite. Everybody seems to be worried about such stomach disorders as ulcers. Even people without a trace of a stomach problem are convinced that one is in their future if they don't take steps to avoid it—or so they claim. Not long ago a man I know told me he was concerned about a sudden weight increase. While he had been heavy for some time, suddenly he began to gain. This weight increase started at about the time he took steps to prevent a recurrent ulcer attack. I wanted to know about this ounce of prevention, and it turned out he was gorging himself on milk, ice cream, puddings! His story is not unique. Many people with ulcers believe they have to consume large amounts of dairy products every day. One treatment for an ulcer may require that certain food be limited—fried foods, for example. But there is no reason to bathe one's gastrointestinal tract in a sea of vanilla ice cream. A quart of ice cream not only may not help an ulcer but it can destroy a waistline. The same holds true for whole milk, heavy cream, puddings, and most other foods associated with ulcer relief. Usually when people fall prey to this myth, they end up overfeeding themselves. If you suspect you have an ulcer and are concerned about what you should and should not eat, see your personal physician. He is in the best position to advise the proper dietary regime for you.

15. *I have a taste for luxury foods, and they are always fattening*. Oh, they are? I guess it depends on what you call a "luxury" food. If it means French pastry to you, then I have to agree. If you are referring to fresh red snapper or a strip of lean veal, I have to disagree. These foods can be very low in calories; it's the cooking and serving methods usually associated with these foods that can be fattening. If you have a yen for red snapper or veal, go right ahead and eat it to your

heart's content—only skip the cream sauce. Exercise your imagination—have the thick, rich sauces in your head.

These are only a few of the more popular myths; there are many, many more. How can you readily distinguish fact from fiction about weight loss? A simple rule is that if a concept raises a barrier between you and your weight loss, it's probably a myth. Keep in mind that you are under no obligation to subscribe to any notion that keeps you from achieving your goal. No rule anywhere on this earth says you must be fat. If you are, and wish to be, dig it! Enjoy it and stop complaining about your weight!

18

"I Need Three Full Meals a Day"

This is a long-standing and deeply held belief that probably causes more problems for people who want to lose weight than all the other popular myths combined. That's why I want to devote a whole chapter to the idea of three full meals a day being an absolute requirement for quick and permanent weight loss.

Three meals a day is a social custom in our culture; it is not a law of nature. Some societies, the Lapps for example, do not have mealtimes at all. A stew pot is kept going over a fire all day long, and as each member of the family feels hungry, he helps himself.

You, as someone who wants to lose weight, are really free to arrange your meal schedule to suit yourself—to eat in a way that works for you. You are free to add or drop meals as you feel necessary. If you are in the habit of skipping one or two meals a day already, my advice to you would be not to change this pattern. You have fewer meals to worry about. A lot of people get themselves into trouble by eating because they feel they should. I lived with this "now or never" syndrome when I was a kid. At times I just was not hungry at six o'clock, but there was always the chance that I might be at nine o'clock. I never did find out, because I never took the chance. It was impressed on me that my mother was supervising a home and family, not an all-night diner. Eating dinner at six o'clock was a now-or-never deal for me. People who believe they will be hungry later usually are. What we believe has a lot to do with what actually happens.

I know people who got themselves into a weight problem by forcing themselves to eat when they were not really hungry. Duncan B. is one. A bachelor in his late twenties, he worked as a salesman. Because he liked sleeping as late as possible in the morning and because he hated messing up the kitchen by cooking for one person, he got into the habit of eating only lunch. At midday, Duncan, who usually had a client with him, would sit down to a substantial lunch. In the evenings, if he felt hungry, he would have a few crackers and a glass of milk. This pattern worked well for Duncan until somebody convinced him he needed three full meals a day. So he started to drag himself out of bed an hour earlier to eat a breakfast of eggs, toast, and bacon; then he would have his usual lunch; and in the evening he would make himself a full dinner of meat, potatoes, vegetables, and a salad. In a few months, he packed on quite a few pounds. All Duncan had to do was return to the eating pattern that had worked before and drop the three-full-meals-a-day pattern that had proved a flop.

Jeanne J., on the other hand, was devoted to the concept of three full meals a day and wanted to stay with it. She loved a complete break in her daily routine at regular intervals. So she had half her normal servings at every meal and dropped desserts and snacks—at least in reality. She treated herself to a few food fantasies every day. This pattern proved to be one that worked for her.

Jan B. was different entirely. She was a dedicated snacker. I do not think Jan can remember the last time she sat down to a "meal" in the true sense of the word. She was a commercial artist who worked at home and kept a weird schedule; that is partly how she learned the snacking style in the first place. When she wanted a break, Jan would knock off for fifteen or twenty minutes to eat. This pattern was not her problem. *What* she snacked on was the trouble. She kept her cabinets well stocked with cookies, cakes, pies, and things like that. When she switched her snack foods to fruits, raw vegetables, and yogurt, her weight problem disappeared.

Jan also discovered that a fifteen- or twenty-minute break did not have to mean eating. She could spend her break acknowledging her worth as a person and as an artist or spend a few minutes fantasizing about a food. Well, Jan is still snacking her way through life, and she is still thin.

Another myth within the three-full-meals-a-day myth is that you *need* a good breakfast under your belt every morning. Maybe you do, but then again, maybe you don't. Attitudes and beliefs about breakfast, as with so many other things, depend on your point of view. The traditional American point of view is the belief in the "hearty breakfast." Some people are comfortable operating within the confines of this tradition, and it works for *them*. Fine. But many people are uncomfortable operating this way, and it does not work for them. This is fine, too. Always keep in mind: it's a matter of viewpoint. Tradition is only one point of view.

The French hold that breakfast should be a roll and a cup of coffee. Anything else, in their eyes, is disgusting and borders on being uncivilized. Yet the traditional French breakfast seems to work. I spent a lot of time traveling with French people when I was in Morocco. I did not see anyone faint in the streets before lunch. The French, with their small breakfast, seemed to function as well as those who start the day with a big breakfast.

The point is: a human being needs a lot less food than is generally realized. Our news media offer any number of examples of people who have survived a lack of food over an incredibly long period of time. Even with a total absence of food, it takes quite a while to starve to death. People are a lot stronger than they give themselves credit for.

I'm saying you have to determine what is right for you;

what works for you is what you want to do. If you're not hungry, do not force yourself to eat just because it seems appropriate or just because of the time of day. Hunger is not governed by the clock or by tradition; it is governed by you. When you want food, you will know it! When or how often you eat is not as important as what and how you eat. One big meal, one small meal, three medium-sized meals, three small meals, or perhaps several small snacks every day may be the pattern that is best for you. What is important is that you eat thin foods, not fat foods; eaten in the thin way, not the fat way. Once you have learned both, then you make the choice.

19

Stories from Successful Learners

There are always more tips to help make taking (and keeping) weight off more successful. The ones listed here come mainly from people I have met who told me their success stories. You will probably think up some shortcuts of your own as time goes by, but these will serve to get you started. As you discover tips for a more successful weight loss, you can always share them with other would-be learners.

1. *Eat off a smaller plate.* This is a great way to create the illusion of having more food when you reduce your serving sizes. The size of the plate is in better proportion to the amount of food you are going to eat. When you cut down on your serving size, the food looks skimpy when you use the standard 10-inch dinner plate.

2. *Drink two glasses of water fifteen or twenty minutes before eating.* Water has no calories, but it is a great filler. Don't just gulp the water. Enjoy it. Treat it as something special. One man told me how he fantasized a glass of water as a tall, creamy vanilla malted. The malted was so good, to his mind, that he wanted it to last. This caused him to linger over the glass of water instead of just gulping it down. With this trick, he learned a new behavior—relaxing with a glass or two of water before dinner—and he ate less. You can also try a

glass of water when you feel you *must* have something to eat. Usually drinking water, coffee, or tea will quiet a hunger pain. And never pass up an opportunity for dream eating. Imagine you are eating something you love when a hunger pain comes along.

3. *You do not have to swallow everything you put in your mouth.* Just chew the food slowly and thoroughly to enjoy the taste. Then take it out of your mouth. If it's not in your stomach, it can't put weight on your hips.

4. *Plan in advance what you will eat.* Each day, sit down and list what you will eat that day or the following day. This will keep you from being caught off guard. You can even plan ahead if you eat out a lot: become a menu collector. Michelle taught me this trick. When I started to learn a new eating behavior, every time we went to a new restaurant she would ask to take a menu as a souvenir. She was always given one (Michelle is much prettier than I am). Each time we planned to go back to a particular restaurant, I would get out the menu and decide in advance what I would have. In the restaurant, I placed my order without looking at the menu. If there is a favorite dish or dessert you simply have to eat, go ahead and have it—but in your head. Sit down and treat yourself to the food via your imagination. As I mentioned earlier, mental eating is a great way to fill up a physical stomach.

5. *Keep yourself busy.* The less you eat, the faster you'll lose weight. There is no way to get around that fact. So you have to fill the time you would otherwise spend eating—after all, you don't want to sit around twiddling your thumbs. Why not take the time to acknowledge your self-worth? Or now that you have some free time, look around you and notice the interesting world you live in. What you do to fill your time, of course, is up to you. It depends on your likes and interests. There must be something you've always wanted to do—play golf, take up a craft, join an organization. What better time than now? When the activity is something you

truly enjoy, you're not going to want to give up that time so you can eat!

6. *Exercise*. If you like sports or enjoy being in motion, an exercise program may assist you in shaking off a few extra pounds. Almost any form of physical activity can help if you want to use it. Consider using your car as little as possible. Walking and bike riding are probably the most painless forms of exercise. And because of the interest in the environment, both are very fashionable these days. A lot of people, I know, believe exercise has to be done regularly. Playing a game of tennis once a month or walking around the block once a week may not yield the terrific results you hoped for. But what about thinking your fat away? There is nothing wrong with mentally exercising your fat cells. If you can picture your fat cells and create enough energy, I truly believe you can burn up calories just by thinking about it. After all, every activity, including thinking, requires us to burn energy.

7. *One picture is worth a thousand words*. Trite but true. Find a picture (or several) of people with great figures. Look for the body you would like to have. Check out magazines, newspapers, maybe even your family album. Paste a picture of your head over the head belonging to the fabulous body. Now that you have a picture of you with a slim figure, put it up. Anywhere—on the refrigerator door, on the bedside table. Just display it so you will have a constant reminder of how you *can* and *will* look if you lose weight.

8. *As your weight drops, get rid of your fat clothes*. Get excited about needing new clothes. Enjoy the anticipation. Until you reach your goal weight, replace your fat discards with a few inexpensive things. As your clothing size decreases, you can remove the larger sizes from your wardrobe without feeling you are wasting money. Give your fat clothes to a charity and enjoy and acknowledge your generosity.

9. *Invest in the new you*. This is probably the strongest, most positive commitment you can make to your future.

When you make an investment, you are saying to yourself in effect, "It's coming, and I'm ready for it." This positive step worked for me. It has also worked for others.

After I set a weight goal for myself, I decided to take a positive step toward it by making an investment in my future. There were no doubts in my mind about shedding those unwanted pounds. They were coming off, and I was going to be prepared for the new me. As I mentioned before, I'm crazy about clothes. Maybe this is because I never had a choice when I was fat. I had to settle for what fit. If I did not care for the design, the color, or the fabric, that was too bad. It was either that or run around in my scrub suit. It looked like a tent, but at one time that was the only thing that fit me.

Once I was thin, I knew I would have a choice. I could pick and choose as I pleased. That, I decided, would be my investment. I would start creating my wardrobe right away. When I reached my goal weight, everything would be ready.

One afternoon, I strolled into a European specialty store and plunked down more money than I could really afford on a pair of slacks. The salesman who waited on me was suspicious, I have to admit; but I said something about a present for a good friend. He was my height, but he weighed about one hundred pounds less. Finally, I just selected a pair of slacks that I liked. As soon as I got home, I hung the slacks up just outside the kitchen door. Every time I was tempted to get something to eat from the kitchen, I would see those slacks. When I was away from home and some tempting bit of food came my way, I would think of those slacks. Thoughts like, "Larry, do you really want to wear those pants? Unless you lose weight, you won't be able to." Just thinking of how much I wanted to wear them was a great assist in keeping me on target.

Clothing is only one example of an investment in your future. If you are disinterested in what you wear, new clothes are not going to help you much. Unless, that is, you are disinterested because of your weight. After you slim down, you may discover that what you wear is very important to you. You will know this when you reach your weight goal.

One man I know invested in tennis lessons. For years he wanted to play the game, but was ashamed to be seen on the courts weighing 243 pounds. "After all," he said, "who wants to watch a clumsy butterball bouncing around the courts? Once I decided the flab was going and going soon, I went over to a tennis club and signed up for lessons four months in the future. Now I had a choice—stay fat and lose the opportunity to do something I really wanted, or lose weight and enjoy a new activity."

Not too long ago, a woman told me that when she was fat she could never bring herself to wear perfume. "There was no rhyme or reason to it," she said. "I just associated perfume with slender, sexy women. It seemed ridiculous for me at my weight to use the stuff. When I decided I was going to knock off my extra weight, I went out and bought a small bottle of perfume. I left it on my dressing table and thought about it constantly. That little bottle became more important to me than food—I really mean that. Every day I would see it while I was dressing for work. As I got thinner, I got more and more excited about using the perfume. Then came the day when I lost the weight I planned to. What a thrill it was to use that perfume! For the first time in ages, I felt so feminine."

Think about something that you can do (or wear) when you lose weight. Start working on it. Having something waiting for the new you—something that is very important to you—will make food even less important in your life.

10. *Have more than one scale in your home.* Keep them around and in sight so you can hop on every time you pass a scale. One in the kitchen, one in the bedroom. This is helpful because you will want to weigh yourself more often than the usual first thing in the morning and last thing at night. Ron Pion made the great suggestion to me that I keep a scale in the office. Why not take a scale to work with you and weigh yourself several times during the day?

11. *Put a mirror on your refrigerator door.* Every time you go to open that door, you can consider how you look now as opposed to how you want to look in the near future.

12. *Tell those who admire and respect you what you are doing.* If you have a nephew, niece, or anyone else who thinks you're just tops, it's human nature for you to want to live up to their expectations. Announce you are planning to lose weight, and your admirer is going to assume you mean exactly what you say. You are going to want to justify that faith and achieve your goal.

Have fun using these hints and suggestions. Have fun discovering your own, too.

20

I Love You—Eat!

Losing weight can be a lot of fun because you will be adopting a new point of view: that learning can be fun and easy. Losing weight can also be a challenge. There is the challenge of creating the new you, which could be one of your highest forms of self-expression. There will also be barriers. Most of the barriers can be easily handled if you are willing to leave them alone. Barriers that block your path are the ones that come from within you. And what you create you can also remove.

One very common barrier you will probably face during the period of your weight loss may come from outside you. Ironically, it is not going to come from those who do not care one way or the other about you or from people who cannot stand you. This barrier is going to come from the people who are closest to you, your family and friends—the very people who love and care about you the most.

You are going to be face to face with any number of friends and relatives who are going to urge you to eat something you do not want. Regardless of how much they believe they are supporting you, they will proudly display a food that will not help you toward your goal. "Just one little piece won't hurt you," they will say. Or, "But I made this just for you. It's your favorite."

These people who want to feed you do love you. In our society, offering food is offering love and approval. Most people who display tempting goodies do so not to hurt or frustrate you, but because they want to show their approval of you. Sometimes an offer of something to eat is just one way of displaying affection. For some people, this is the only way they know. An offer of food shows their desire to please. Rejection of food can be misinterpreted as a rejection of love. Notice I said it *can be*. It does not have to be. There is a way to protect yourself and your personal goals and still allow your close friends and relatives to support you and your goals.

I have worked out a scenario for this situation. It covers most of the arguments for eating a food you do not want. Go over it carefully. Make changes to suit your personal situation. Practice saying it many times. Here's where your tape recorder can be a big help. Say the words so they sound convincing. True conviction on your part is very important because as soon as someone offering food thinks that you're kidding or are insincere, they will come on even stronger. The idea is to change what they are saying to you so that it supports you and them.

The time is the not too distant past. My weight loss program is going along nicely, and I'm pleased, even thrilled, with my progress. An invitation to dinner comes from one of my favorite relatives, Aunt Elly. She has a justly deserved family reputation for her pecan schnecken. This is not just any pecan schnecken; this is a work of art. The dough is baked to a rich golden brown. The filling is soft melted brown sugar mixed with dozens of crushed pecans and held together with lots of butter. When the schnecken are being baked, the aroma floats out from the kitchen throughout her house.

I like Aunt Elly's schnecken as much as anybody. I also

know I will be offered a piece, and the last thing I want to do is physically eat that schnecken. How am I going to refuse the pastry and make it stick? And not risk hurting Aunt Elly's feelings?

Dinner is over, and it's time for dessert. Sure enough, Aunt Elly vanishes into the kitchen and comes back carrying her pride and joy—a plate of pecan schnecken. Swirls of golden dough filled with that thick mixture of pecans and brown sugar and swimming in honey. Beaming with pleasure, Aunt Elly starts to serve me the biggest one on the plate.

LARRY: No schnecken for me, thank you, Aunt Elly.

ELLY: Did I hear right? No schnecken?

L: That's right. I'll pass it by. You have a piece, though.

E: I never heard you say no to a piece of my schnecken. What's come over you? Are you sick or something?

L: No, I feel fine. In fact, I feel better than ever.

E: Then why don't you want a piece of schnecken? It's nice and fresh. I baked it this afternoon just for you.

L: Yes, I know you did, and I do appreciate it. But just looking at it and inhaling that aroma satisfies me. I don't have to eat it to enjoy it.

E: Just looking at it? What's gotten into you? Usually you have three or four pieces.

L: I've learned a new behavior that allows me to enjoy foods without having to eat them. I *imagine* I'm eating them. Right now, I can sit here and pretend I'm eating a schnecken and be satisfied.

E: Pretend you're eating something! That's the silliest thing I've ever heard. And, Larry, from you of all people! Stop teasing me, and eat.

L: I'm not teasing you, I'm very serious. I can pretend I'm eating anything I want and have the feeling that I'm eating it. It strikes you as silly because it's a new idea. But not too long ago, the idea of going to the moon was silly, too. [*Almost everybody finds new ideas, new be-*

haviors, and new foods odd, even silly, the first time around. Once a new viewpoint is learned, the idea isn't silly any more.]

E: Larry, what are you up to?

L: I don't know whether I told you or not, but I'm going to lose weight. I started to learn a new eating behavior about three months ago, and I've already lost close to twenty pounds. I'm so pleased with my progress! If I have a piece of schnecken it would only slow down my progress.

E: You on a diet? Again? You've been on eight diets in the last six years and none of them worked! Forget this silly notion and have a piece of schnecken. Why waste your time trying to lose weight? You can't help being hefty—it comes from my side of the family. We've always been heavy—but we eat good. That's the important thing.

L: I know I didn't achieve my goal during my other attempts to lose weight, but I'm doing wonderfully this time. I've already lost nearly twenty pounds, and if my weight was something I couldn't help, I don't believe I would have slimmed down as much as I have. I stopped accusing your side of the family for my weight problem. My eating habits made me fat, not my heredity. Our family is off the hook for that one.

E: I guess *you have* lost some weight. You know, I thought you looked a little tired and drawn when you came in. It's because of that weight you lost. If you look this way after almost twenty pounds, you'll look like death warmed over after forty pounds. You mark my words. Have some schnecken and stop this nonsense.

L: It's not nonsense at all—it's wonderful. You probably think I look tired and drawn because you've always known me padded with fat. You're not used to the new me, that's all. In a little while you'll get used to it. Why don't you have a piece of schnecken yourself?

E: Forget about me. I made this for you so you could have something you like. I want to make you happy.

L: You *have* made me happy. Just by thinking of me in such a nice way, you make me very happy. Would you like to do something else for me? Something I really want and need? Something that will make me happy?

E: Certainly! Just ask. That's what relatives are for. If you can't ask your family, who can you ask?

L: I know that, and that's why I'm coming to you. I'd like your support—I need your help and support in this weight loss program of mine. It means a lot to me that I succeed, and you are one of the few people who is in a position to help me along. Anybody can make me a schnecken, even a stranger, but only someone who really cares can give me help and support.

E: Well, if you put it that way, I guess so. But still and all, what's a visit to me without a piece of my pecan schnecken?

L: I knew I could depend on you. Thank you. But while we're on the subject, have you ever thought about why I visit you?

E: Why you visit me? I don't understand what you mean.

L: I want to know if you know why I visit you. You said, "What's a visit without a piece of my schnecken?" The truth is that I don't come to see you because you make the best schnecken in the world. I come to see you because I love you and enjoy being with you—you, not your schnecken. Even if you were the worst cook in the world, which you are not, I'd still look forward to spending an evening with you. But I come to see you, and you alone. You are more important to me than your excellent food.

E: Well, dear, I guess I see your point, and thank you for those nice words, but ever since you were little you loved my schnecken. This is all a surprise to me, and it takes a little getting used to. [*Another new behavior that is awkward at first.*]

L: I know when I was little, I was always eating your schnecken. But when I was little I also loved riding my tricycle. Adults do different things from little kids, that's all. Remember when I was little, how I hated cucumbers? I always picked them out of the salads you made?

E: Indeed I do. That was an awful habit. Putting your fingers in your food like that.

L: Did you notice this evening I ate the cucumbers? I didn't pick them out of the salad?

E: I guess I didn't.

L: I ate them and enjoyed them. I've learned to like cucumbers since I've been on this program. Especially nice juicy fresh ones from somebody's garden.

E: It's about time you learned something about good food. I told you years ago cucumbers were good for you. But what am I going to do with this schnecken? If you don't eat it, nobody else will. I hate to see it go to waste.

L: That's no problem, if you're really worried about it. There's the hospital you love donating your time to. They're having their annual cake sale tomorrow afternoon. You know they'd love to have your schnecken as a donation. Come on, we can go over there right now and donate the pastry in your name. That will solve everything. I won't eat it, it won't go to waste, and the money raised will go to help a good cause.

Chances are you will not have to explain your case beyond this point. It's a good idea to know an organization in the neighborhood that will accept gifts of food. You will not have far to look. Almost any hospital, service club, nursing home, orphanage, or religious group will be pleased to have donations of food.

By applying your point of view like this, you can establish and maintain a number of points. You know you have not lost weight in the past, but this time you have and mean to continue. You intend to maintain your success. You, personally, believe you look and feel better since your weight loss, and believe you will look and feel even better when all the excess weight is gone.

Another thing you have done is to establish the fact that you like the person for him- or herself, and not for the food. By the way, should it turn out that you see certain people not because you like them but only because you like their food, why are you wasting time visiting with them? If food that you do not want to eat is the only attraction, you can put your time to better use. When you tell people you come to see them for their personality alone, you are truly expressing love. You have paid a sincere and deep compliment.

More important, you have effectively handled what used to be the old pressure to eat unwanted, unnecessary food by turning the tables. You have asked someone who cares for you to help you. You have let it be known that you want and need their support. When there is an emotional bond between two people, a request of this sort is very difficult to refuse. People who care for you want the best for you; they want to back your efforts, they want to see you achieve your goals. At the same time, you are supporting the other person. You have let them know how much you care for them. You care for them because they are who they are. You are giving them self-esteem.

Unless you lead a completely antisocial life, and very few of us do, you are going to need some help and support from your family and friends. Spread the word about your project and ask that they back you up. There is nothing to be ashamed of. Wanting to look your best and feel your best is something to be proud of. Also, tell them that you will support them in *their* activities; that you are willing to help them reach *their* goals.

You're going to need help and support, too, when someone other than yourself is in charge of the cooking. Your parents, your spouse, your roommate, whoever does the cooking will have to know that you will be handling certain foods in new ways. But be sure to explain that you do not hold the family cook responsible for your weight problem.

Anyone wanting to lose weight, no matter how dedicated they are, still does not have the right to impose their new eating style on other people. If your regular table companions want baked potatoes with sour cream, let them have the potatoes and support their enjoyment. Support them in their desires as they support you. All you can do is make it plain (use the Aunt Elly scenario, if necessary) that you are not interested in eating baked potatoes with sour cream.

Letting others know that you are not going to insist that they follow your eating style is important. Many would-be thin people help themselves fail by insisting that everyone they live with move in the same direction. This can cause resentment, and there is no faster way to turn off support and the desire to help than by causing those who can give it to resent you.

Do not be surprised or hurt if those you live with still want to eat cookies and salted nuts. They are not trying to make life miserable for you. Living with this sort of food within easy reach will be good practice for you. As you proceed toward your goal, the rest of the world is going on as before. Bakery owners will not cover the display window just because you walk by, supermarket managers will not block off the snack aisles just because you shop there, and the coffee wagon in your office will not disappear.

Not everyone you associate with needs or wants to lose weight. You do, so you have the responsibility of establishing your own eating pattern. You eat what works for you, and let others eat what works for them. Enjoy the power you will feel for successfully negotiating this part of your life. Acknowledge yourself for your achievement, and acknowledge all those who have supported you.

21

Maintenance

Once you have reached the weight you want to be, then what?
What do you do to stay where you are? Somewhere along the
line you will want to stop losing weight. It is entirely possible
that you will decide that you are just a bit too thin. I was like
that. Once I slimmed down, I found I looked too gaunt. That
was easy to remedy. I just gained two or three pounds. That
did the trick.

Maintenance is nothing more than applying the new behavior you have learned. With a few modifications, that is.
You have to experiment with different foods and find out
what works for you. Today, I eat whatever I want. I still eat
pecan pie in reality. The only difference is that I do not eat
it as often as I used to. Perhaps once or twice a month I'll
have a piece. This pattern works for me and suits my goal—
to stay thin. I know very well, that if I ate a piece of pecan
pie every evening those pounds would come creeping back on.

To find your own level, try different foods and check back
with your scale. A lot of weight checks, the more the better,
is the only way of knowing which foods work and which do
not. If you have pastry several days in a row and then step
on the scale and see a few pounds that were not there before,
you know pastry is not working. Right now, I make a point

of weighing myself twice a day—first thing in the morning and the last thing at night.

Try different foods in different quantities and see what happens. Spaghetti once a week may not matter. On the other hand, it may. You'll never know unless you try. Keep in mind that you have a choice now—your old eating style or your new one. You know what happened when you used the old style. Now you know what the new one will achieve.

Apply your newly learned eating behavior and don't forget self-praise and fantasy eating.

What are you going to praise yourself about? Your weight loss? Certainly there is nothing wrong with that, but after a while you may find it boring. Remember when I was losing weight, I said I buttonholed everybody in the hospital and told them how I was doing? After a while, this got dull, even for me. Doing and saying the same thing over and over again can get very tiresome.

We have all met people who can talk about nothing but their ailments. Nobody likes to hear about disease and sickness all the time. The same is true for the opposite. We have all no doubt met people who are into health fads. Listening to the benefits of sea salt and unrefined sugar can get tiring too. The same is true for weight loss. It really is not the only positive aspect of your life. Keep building up your assets and your positive points. Praise yourself for these things as well as your weight loss. Keep on learning, and doing, and experiencing. Make sure you keep yourself interested in all kinds of experiences.

I stay excited about my new eating behaviors by staying excited about all the new foods I have learned to eat. And can these foods be ever exciting! Most of us once learned to look at salad as "rabbit food." Supposedly, there is nothing enjoyable or different about eating a salad. But a salad can be fun—it can be a far-out experience—a fact I learned from a former comedian named Richard Simmons.

Dick used to weigh 268 pounds; he now weighs 135 pounds

and owns a combination exercise spa/salad bar in Los Angeles. He calls the spa the Anatomy Asylum and the salad bar the Ruffage. Just from the names, you can see what a fun guy Dick is. He greets his customers warmly, does a few ballet steps, and makes a few comments about their weight. He has a sharp sense of humor, and his alert gaze misses nothing.

Picture yourself walking into a salad bar designed to look like a cave with a white-on-white decor. Dick Simmons, a slightly built man wearing leotards, leaps over to you and does his ballet steps. Then he gives your figure a shrewd, professional gaze. If your backside is too well padded, he may say gently, "My dear, the chairs are very comfortable. You didn't have to bring your own seat cushion!"

And this different approach does not stop at the door. As you wander over to the mouth-watering salad bar to choose from the wide selection of salads and dressings, Dick often appears again. As you pile your plate high with goodies, he may say wryly, "I see you're having our favorite, 'mounds of everything.' " Or, "Are you feeding your family?"

But the salads are just as much fun as Dick Simmons himself. An incredible sight is his 25-foot salad. Yes, that's right, 25 feet. From this fantastic spread you hunt and pick out your favorite slenderizers. The bed is crisp, fresh spinach and butter lettuce. Artistically laid across the bed are some thirty-five "munchies," as Dick calls them. Along the 25 feet of delicious eating you will find such things as carrots, celery, sweet red peppers, radishes, red and white cabbage, red onions, scallions, cauliflower, zucchini, cucumber, chick-peas, beets, tuna, and tomatoes. All of this can be laced with a wide selection of low-calorie dressings that Dick has developed. Many have a cottage cheese or yogurt base. There are lemon, mushroom, apple, garlic, and cucumber dressings. All are rich and creamy. And to top this off, Dick offers walnuts, raisins, parsley, and poppy seeds.

Before I lost weight, I would never have gone to the Ruffage, and I would have missed out on a lot of fun. Now, every time I am in Los Angeles I can't wait to eat there because I have a good time.

I realize not everyone has a restaurant like the Ruffage close by, but there is nothing stopping you from creating your own fun. Dick Simmons offers just one way to have a good time. There are other ways with food that are equally thrilling. Give expression to your creativity and make your own enjoyment.

The pleasures of new foods are not your only assets. Every day we all do something that is good and deserving of credit. I wake up in the morning I ask myself what it will be and how it will happen. A sense of excitement comes from this anticipation. Each day becomes an adventure. I cannot wait to get going so I can discover a reason for self-praise.

Right now, you might be saying to yourself, "What's so special about my life? I'm just an ordinary person with a home and a family." Nobody, in my opinion, is ordinary. Each of us is unique. And nobody leads an ordinary, uneventful life unless they convince themselves that they do. Everything we do has two sides, the negative and the positive. Far too often, we concentrate on the negative.

Let's pretend you have been asked by your child's teacher to help with a class outing. Okay, shepherding a bunch of kids around can be a hassle. At the end of the day, your reaction could very well be a negative one: "My day was lousy!" You chased after twenty-five kids. One of them was sick on the bus. Another one lost a mitten. But it is possible to see this as an accomplishment, something worthy of self-praise: "It was a good day. I was able to answer their questions. I was able to point out interesting things to the kids. Nobody was left behind."

So you see, no matter how or where we live, things happen every day that allow us to say, "I contributed in a positive

way. I accomplished something. I am worth something!"
This is what self-praise and a feeling of self-worth are all
about—continually adding to our list of positive features.

More about fantasy eating. It is a very valuable behavior
and can help you greatly in maintaining your weight loss.
Sometimes when we learn new behavior, our tastes change.
You may find foods that you loved when you were fat and
cannot stand now that you are thin. Tastes change like everything else. When I was heavy I was crazy about graham
crackers and milk. A big bowl of mashed crackers and lot of
milk—a super snack. Now I can't think of anything more
disgusting. It just does not appeal to me any more.

You will probably find that many fat foods still appeal to
you. I can still flip over pecan pie. And I am not about to
give it up. But I have learned a new, weightless way to eat it.
Oh, sure, I could have a slice for dessert every evening after
dinner. There is nothing stopping me. And there will be nothing stopping you from enjoying your favorite foods in this
manner.

I also know that by having a slice of pie every evening for
dessert I am not going to stay on target. More than anything
else I want to stick to my purpose, and assume you do too.
There will be foods that do not fit in with your goal when
eaten in reality. Foods which, however much they contradict
your goal, you do not want to give up. Well, go right ahead
and eat them—in your mind. And make a big deal out of it.

Several times a week I imagine I am eating a piece of pecan
pie. I don't just eat it. First I get a good fix on what I look
like—where I am, what I am wearing—then I zero in on the
pie itself. Usually it is a 9-inch pie. The edge of the crust has
been twisted into curlicues. Oh, yes, the edge of the crust is
perfectly ruffled. The filling is a rich, dark amber brown. As
I turn the pie every which way, the light catches the golden
highlights. Each pecan is perfect. No broken or bruised nuts.

Then I inhale the aroma. That heavy, sweet scent. Brown
sugar mixed with fresh butter, and held together with dark

corn syrup. Next, I imagine I'm cutting a slice and putting it on a plate. All of this I do *slowly*.

There is no hurry! No one is going to take this pie away from me. I want to enjoy every aspect of the pie, not just the taste. The sight and the aroma are important, too. Once I have done this, I am ready for a taste. Slowly I take my mental fork and cut off a piece. Not a big piece, but not a small one either. Just a normal, average-size piece. I put the piece in my mouth and let it melt there. The filling slowly glides across my taste buds and down my throat, leaving behind the sense of the rich and the delicious. I chew each pecan to a fine paste, mixed together with whatever flaky crust remains in my mouth. All this I swallow—slowly and deliberately.

Sometimes I finish the entire slice of my make-believe pie; other times I have only a few bites. It depends on how hungry I am. Whether or not I have something to drink depends on my mood, too. Occasionally I have a tall, cold glass of milk. In my head, of course. The really great thing about imaginary eating is that *you* decide what you are going to have. And when. And how much. When I treat myself to fantasy food, I am pleasing one person—me. The same applies to you. The goodie is for your pleasure alone.

Every now and again I get the urge for a really rich dessert that I do not want to eat in reality. Satisfaction is only a fantasy away. I take myself on a mental tour of my favorite New York bakeries. Why not come along with me and visit a few super places for rich desserts?

22

Fantasies on My Mind

My favorite fattening fantasies take place in New York City because the Big Apple is home to some of the most incredible bakeries. I love sweets; I flip over desserts, even if now I am more likely to do so with my mind than with my mouth. Depending on my mood, I am likely to stop off in one of three places. Miss Grimble's, famed for cheese cake; Kron Chocolatier, for the fabulous things they do with chocolate; or Bonté's, known for classical French pastry. All three shops are in the same area, the exciting, luxurious silk-stocking district. On our tour, I'll show you around and describe the goodies for you. I think you will enjoy these places as much as I do, and you will want to keep coming back. And you can, you can keep coming as often as you want without lifting a finger or gaining an ounce. Let your mind do the traveling and the eating.

Okay, why not settle back into your favorite place for fantasizing. Get your body into a comfortable position and let your muscles hang loose. Decide what you will be wearing. Decide how you will get to New York. Every now and again, I like to imagine a slow cross-country drive in my car. Once in New York, our first stop will be on Madison Avenue, at Miss Grimble's, the home of the most fabulous cheese cake imaginable. If you are a cheese cake freak, as I am, this is where you want to hang out.

As we walk into the shop, the first thing you will see is the simple decor. Pearly gray walls and an imitation brick floor. Scattered along the walls are framed magazine and newspaper articles about the shop. But this simple background is the perfect setting for the cheese cake gems that are on display in the black-and-white-check showcases. Any kind of cheese cake you want is here—raspberry, chocolate marble, lemon. All with a thick cream-cheese base and a crumb crust.

Let's pretend that one of the co-owners, Lynn, a charming, friendly woman, has invited us into her office for a cup of coffee and a piece of cheese cake. How about raspberry? The cheese cake itself is rich and creamy—a delicate shade of off-white. Laced through its creamy consistency are swirls upon swirls of fresh raspberry. The aroma of the bright red berries surrounds you. Pick up your fork and take a bite. There is no need to chew, because the cake is so soft. Let the cake stay in your mouth and melt slowly so it can wash across your taste buds and down your throat. Sweet, isn't it? Smooth, too. Just delicious. If you would like to finish the piece, go right ahead, but remember, we are going to make two more stops. You don't want to be too full to enjoy the complete tour.

Our second stop is also on Madison Avenue—the fabulous chocolate shop called the Kron Chocolatier owned and operated by Tom and Diane Kron, who are waiting for us. Their shop is on the second floor. As we go in, you will see a nondescript flight of stairs, we walk along a rather drab hallway. While the stairs and hallway are not luxurious, the aroma is. What an enticing first impression your nose will have—the scent of deliciously "brewing" chocolate. As we walk through the door, you will see a tray of chocolate-covered fresh strawberries or raspberries. The Krons offer these treats to all who visit their shop. Try one. They are delicious. In the front of the shop is a large window overlooking Madison Avenue.

Tom and Diane have dozens of plants here to give the shop a garden look. In the back is another large window that looks into the workroom.

Tom and Diane work from an old family recipe that calls for cocoa butter and powdered chocolate. Because they do not use much sugar, their candy is unusually crispy. Their dark, light, and white chocolates have no artificial flavors or colorings. Everything, including the liqueurs, is real.

But it is not only the flavor and quality of the chocolate that makes Kron's so unique, it is also what Tom and Diane do with their product. They design and produce chocolate sculptures. A current favorite is a torso of a nude woman—it is all solid chocolate. But you can also get a chocolate foot, or even chocolate letters to spell out messages. One of my favorite hostess gifts is candy letters to spell out "Thanks." And not too long ago, I ordered two chocolate breasts for a friend of mine who considers himself quite a connoisseur of the female bosom.

With so much to choose from, it is hard to decide. Why not get ourselves into a mood for math? Let's have a solid chocolate ruler. In light chocolate. Yes, it is a regular twelve-inch ruler and marked just like any ordinary ruler you might have around your house. Of course, if you prefer, the ruler can be had in dark or white chocolate. The choice is yours. Break off an inch and pop it in your mouth. This is another food that does not have to be chewed. Letting it melt in your mouth makes the taste last longer. Of course, if you are a chocolate chewer, the Kron's product is so crispy that chewing is a treat in itself.

Again, if you wish, we can finish the whole twelve-inch ruler. Savor the taste and smoothness of the candy all you want. But there is another stop that we are going to make. Do you have room enough for cheese cake, chocolate, *and* French pastry? You be the judge of your capacity. We can say good-bye to Tom and Diane Kron now and leave.

Since it is such a beautiful day, why don't we walk over to Bonté's on Third Avenue. The walk along the crosstown blocks can be very interesting. Some lovely townhouses and apartment buildings line the streets. Many of the famous celebrities and socialites that we read about every day live in this neighborhood. Maybe we will spot one or two. Whenever I make this fantasy trip to New York, I include a celebrity or two.

On more than one occasion the Bonté Patisserie has been rated the best French pastry shop in New York. The owner of the shop, Maurice Bonté, has used red and white to decorate. Two large showcases line the walls, and there are two hanging showcases. To add a touch of Paris, M. Bonte displays a photograph of the President of the French Republic. Maurice is a true Frenchman. To him, baking is an art, and he can be seen in the shop dressed in a chef's uniform. He takes an active part in the creation of delicious éclairs, cream puffs, and napoleons, not to mention my special favorite. It is called succulent, and I think we should try a piece.

Succulent is a high, handsome, golden cake. Maurice creates this taste treat by using alternating layers of crisp meringue, gold genoise cake, and Grand Marnier butter cream sharpened with bitter Seville orange rinds. And, *voilà*, a masterpiece, a work of art that would not disgrace the Louvre.

And we can have a piece. What I like to do with this cake after I put a piece in my mouth is to separate the layers. I use my tongue to do this. The genoise cake is usually first. Then I like to mix in the butter cream. And finally the meringue. Succulent is just that—there is no other way to describe it. Sweet, but not too sweet because of the orange rinds. Even as you chew each mouthful, you can feel hundreds of calories ooze down your throat. Moist but not soggy. Full but not heavy. Succulent is every pastry dream come true.

Once I have taken myself on a dessert tour of New York, I am satisfied. On some trips I eat more than on others. In some fantasies, I stop at just one place; in others, I visit all three. But no matter how I arrange my mental schedule, I stay until I am satisfied.

And the nice thing about eating this way is you can take this fantasy tour anytime you want. Your mental creation can be made as elaborate as you wish. You can create conversations, shopping excursions to the big stores, anything you want.

I have set the stage for you. But I did not want to cramp your imagination by giving you the whole plot and the whole script, because you can do that. The details are the most fun, and I hope you can please yourself.

23

The Next Generation

I am frequently invited to talk with groups of people. The
topic usually involves learning facilitation and the process of
change. The subjects can vary from sexual satisfaction to
parenting skills to, you guessed it, eating the right "weigh."
At the end of the talk, I try to include a question-and-answer
session. If the topic has been weight problems, someone in
the audience is almost certain to ask, "How can I teach my
children to be thin?"

That is a good question. A child who learns to be thin has
an excellent chance of not having a fat problem. Of course,
there is no guarantee that a child, at some later date, will not
learn to be fat. But the odds in favor of thinness are pretty
good. Since you have lived in the fat world, you know what
a drag it can be. You don't want your offspring to develop
the problem you faced. That is why I am including a few tips
that can help. By keeping them in mind, you can teach your
children some valuable lessons about food. Most of these
hints come from parents who have found them useful in
teaching their children.

1. *As far as possible, teach your children to associate food
with the need to eat.* I realize there have to be certain times
set aside for meals, but if your child is not hungry at the

regular eating time, do not force large amounts of food. You might consider keeping a selection of easy-to-prepare thin foods like vegetables and fruits on hand to serve as snacks when a hunger pain occurs after the meal is over.

2. *Start off with small helpings.* Many parents make the mistake of overloading a kid's plate and then they get annoyed when all the food is not eaten. By starting off with a bit of this and a bit of that, the child can always come back for seconds. I know a lot of parents feel guilty about putting a small amount of food in front of their children, but they need not. Keep in mind that children do not have adult-sized stomachs and therefore have a lesser capacity for food anyway.

3. *If your child does not want to finish his food, accept the fact.* Do not use a philosophy of "take all you want, but eat all you take." This can lead to learning to eat everything in sight. No child willingly starves; when food is refused, it is because there is no desire to eat. If you do not like to throw food away, reduce the serving sizes for the child. A lecture about people who are starving somewhere in the world is not the way to teach a child to be a thin adult. Opening a chapter of the Clean Plate Club in your home might be asking for a fat kid.

4. *Do not feel slighted if your child refuses food, even if it is something you pride yourself on.* Having done my own cooking for a number of years, I know how much work can go into preparing a meal. Good food takes thought, time, and effort; and when we make this kind of an investment, we would like a little appreciation. This is human nature, but if your child refuses a dish you spent hours preparing, he is not doing so because he dislikes you. He might be refusing food because he is not hungry. Don't take it personally when someone says "No, thank you" to food, even if it *is* your famous roast beef.

5. *Do not put your child on the spot about food.* This is an extension of the previous suggestion, but it is so easy to fall

into the routine of "Mommy made this just for you, so why not have a little?" In a situation like this, what is the kid going to say? Children are very anxious to please, so naturally the food, if pushed, will be accepted. There is no reason to make a child feel guilty for not wanting food.

6. *Never use food as a reward or punishment.* Food is an essential requirement for life just as oxygen is. Remove either one for a long enough period of time and life ceases. Yet parents who would never dream of saying to a child who has done something wrong, "Because you did that, you're going to bed without oxygen tonight," will casually announce, "No dinner for you tonight." Parents who would never think of rewarding their children with an extra whiff of oxygen will bubble, "You did such a great job! This calls for a dish of ice cream."

I am not saying that children do not need guidance and rewards; I am saying that food should not enter the picture. Guidance can be just as effective, probably more so, if it involves loss of a privilege. Rather than withholding food, withhold television or something like that. Even better, model for them the behavior you would like. Rewards, too, are more effective if they involve something special and out of the ordinary. Don't make eating into something special. The next time you want to reward your child, instead of opening the refrigerator door, why not suggest a trip to the movies, a new toy—something like that?

7. *Teach your children to use their imagination.* Rewards do not have to be material to be valuable. Mental rewards are just as effective. Kids have great imaginations, and they should be encouraged to develop their creative mind skills. Make sure your child knows that purposeful daydreaming is an approved activity.

8. *Do not use food to repair a shattered ego.* All kids have problems, tragedies, and crises; usually adults see these upsets as small stuff and are inclined to fluff them off with a glass of milk and a few cookies. One of these days, your

child is going to come home in tears about something. This could be anything from a scraped knee to a tearful confession of, "I tripped over a chair in the lunchroom, and all the kids laughed at me!" However minor these problems seem to an adult, to a child they might as well be the end of the world. A sympathetic shoulder, an inviting lap, and a secure pair of arms will heal the bruised ego much faster than cookies.

9. *Let your child see you enjoying thin foods.* This way you can be a model for your child to learn from. Kids are great little imitators and want to do what they see their parents doing. If they see you enjoying carrot sticks during your afternoon coffee break, they will want to munch along, too. Talk to them about these foods. Discuss the colors, the aromas, and the feel of thin foods. Kids are very sensitive to adult emotions, and if you are excited about thin foods, they will sense this and get enthusiastic themselves.

10. *Above all, praise your child for his abilities and accomplishments.* Let him know he is worthy, especially if he is on the tubby side right now. Chances are he is getting some teasing from the other kids about his weight. What he needs from you is help in building up his self-esteem.

These suggestions should help you teach your child to be thin. The idea is to expose children to the concept that we eat to live; we do not live to eat. Once this concept is learned, more than likely food will be used and not abused by the next generation.

24

One Woman's Story—An Example of a Tape

Because making a biographical tape is a new experience for many of you, I am including a transcript of a tape. When I first met Laura Anderson, she weighed 188 pounds; now she weighs 168 pounds and is still losing. When I reviewed Laura's tape, I was struck by the fact that her story is a perfect example for you to learn from. Before you start making your own tape, read Laura's story. I think you will get some ideas for the points you'll want to make on your own tape. Of course your story will not be exactly like Laura's. Nor should it be—you are unique; therefore your background and experiences are unique. I have made a number of parenthetical remarks to emphasize what Laura brought out. Notice that Laura uses a natural, informal style when speaking.

"I am a forty-five-year-old woman, a wife, a mother, and a registered nurse. I have been overweight since early childhood and have been on diet after diet since my early teenage years. [*Laura states her problem.*] How did my problem come about? I can only give theories. When I was a little girl, a very young child, I understand that I was willing to eat anything that was put into my mouth. That made me the good little girl, as opposed to my sister who used to spit out food and give the family lots of problems. [*An early learning experience—rewarded for eating all the food put in front of her*.] Whether that was an influencing factor, I really don't know. When I was five, almost six years old, my family left Nazi Germany and fled to the United States. Up to that time, I believe I had been a happy-go-lucky little child. There was a lot of uncertainty in the family. My father was a doctor, and he had to study hard for over a year before he was able to take the state board exams successfully. After he took the state boards, he tried to find a place for the family to live. During that time I was farmed out to an aunt and uncle in Richmond, Virginia.

"I remember being dreadfully unhappy there. My aunt and uncle had a son and a daughter. The son was the same age as I, and the daughter a little bit older, and there was a lot of unrest in that family. A lot of sibling rivalry, and I felt very uncomfortable and terribly homesick for my family. When finally after about three months my father came to pick me up, I followed him like a little lost sheep. We went to our new home in upstate New York by train, and we had to make a stop. My father brought me to the ladies' room, and he went into the men's room. I came out first, and did not find him, and my father could hear me crying from the men's room. I remember this experience very vividly, and to this day I have a dread of being lost.

"My third theory, and maybe the one that holds the most weight, is that I believe I have a learning disability which was never detected because that type of thing was not thought of in those days. My oldest daughter has a learning disability which manifests itself in not being able to spell, and consequently, not being able to read well, and I remember, looking back on my school days, that I had trouble with spelling (and still do to this day), and I was a slow learner as opposed to my sister, who was very bright and a very quick learner. I know, or feel, that that gave me a tremendous lack of self-confidence, and I feel that a great deal of my problem stems from the fact that I lacked self-confidence. [*Here Laura is showing evidence of low self-esteem.*]

"I am very concerned with the way I look. I do not like being fat. I do enjoy getting dressed up, and it is difficult to find clothing in a large size, particularly since I am quite short and short-waisted, so it's doubly hard for me to find a dress that really looks nice on me. I also would like to improve the way I feel. I fatigue very easily. I've had back problems. Problems with a degenerated disc, and I am certain that that would improve if I could take off some weight. I'm also aware of a number of heart problems in the family. My own father passed away from a heart attack, and consequently I know that as far as my health is concerned, it would be much better to lose weight. [*These are liabilities that could be turned into assets.*]

"I started dieting as a teen-ager and was never very successful at it. [*Past failures that can hinder future progress.*] I was always very unsure of myself as a teen-ager. I seldom dated. I made friends with girls quite easily, but never had any good relationship with a boy. I was quite active in high school. I was in clubs. I was editor of the yearbook. President of the library club. [*Laura does have positive abilities, but perhaps she overlooked her strong points.*] My best relationships were always with girls as opposed to boys. That made me unhappy both with myself and with . . . Well, just unhappy in general. At the age of eighteen I went into nursing school, and I was very overweight and still very unsure of myself at that point. [*Laura continued to keep her problem around. She continued to identify with failure and suffer low self-esteem.*]

"After six months of nursing school I was not doing a good job as far as my scholastic work went, and I was put on probation. This made me yet more unsure and very apprehensive. After the six months were over, though, we started to go onto the floor and begin patient care, and I quickly found that I was very good in that sphere of nursing, that I related very well to patients and they to me, and that gave me a great deal of self-confidence. There was much less learning, so to speak, book learning, and I found nursing school much easier from that point on, and I even began to do better as far as scholastic work was concerned. [*Assets are being uncovered.*] That maybe goes back to the learning disability problem and the lack of self-confidence that gave me. However, to this day I think my nursing experiences were probably the most positive experiences that I've had in the way of enforcing self-confidence. [*Laura can learn to use these assets well.*]

"I feel that I am a good nurse. Patients relate well to me and I relate well to my patients, and that always gives me a good feeling. I enjoy nursing. Whenever I start a new job, I always feel very apprehensive, and perhaps don't do as good a job as I do after a certain period of time when I feel that I know the ropes and feel confident in myself. But I don't feel that there's ever been a case in which I haven't done a good job and in which my employers and my patients weren't satisfied with me, and I was always very happy in most of my working situations. [*More assets. When we really start looking for them, they can pile up quickly.*]

"My father passed away almost immediately after I graduated from nursing school, and that was a very traumatic experience for me. I left New York City, where I had graduated from nursing school and was then working, and went upstate New York to stay with my mother and help her to sell our home and tie up loose ends. I stayed with her for about six to eight months. Then my mother and I moved to New York City together and shared an apartment. I continued working and at that point started doing public health nursing in New York City. I enjoyed public health nursing very much, and found a lot of confidence in myself. There was a lot of work that I had to do on my own, and I felt that I was doing a very good job. I started to lose some weight at this point in my life also. [*Life started to work for Laura, and she was taking responsibility.*] However, I was dieting. I was dieting with the help of amphetamines. And I did start to have a little bit of a social life. I dated occasionally.

"About this time I met a young man that I really liked very much, and I really thought that I was in love with him, and we dated occasionally. Started dating maybe a little more than occasionally and then, all of a sudden after maybe six months or so, I found out that he was going out with his secretary at work, and he no longer asked me out for dates, and I was very, very miserable and unhappy over that situation. Right about this time, my mother had been dating an old family friend, a doctor who had gone to school with my dad, and they became serious. And I would say maybe two years after my father passed away, my mother remarried, and this didn't help my self-confidence very much. My mother remarrying, and here I was minus a boy friend. [*Laura is putting up barriers.*]

"Anyway, at this point I went to San Francisco with a girl friend, and that's probably the best thing I ever did for myself, because I was very happy in San Francisco. I really loved it there, and this friend of mine had been living there and had already developed a very nice group of friends. Most of them were young people she met through the temple, and we went regularly to meetings and outings, and my social life became quite good. I had a very nice job in the outpatient clinic of the hospital. And I was really happy with that job. I started losing weight and went down quite a bit, always with the help of amphetamines. [*A possible barrier. In order to lose weight, Laura needs amphetamines.*]

"In fact, at that point I was taking quite a large dose of amphetamines, and after I had been in San Francisco about a year, I met my husband and we started dating quite steadily, and I continued to lose weight, and I got down to about 123 pounds. I looked very good when we got married. [*Life was working. Dieting worked. It seemed like everything started*

to look good.] At that point I stopped taking the amphetamines, and I don't know why I stopped. My husband was
going to school, and we moved to Ann Arbor, Michigan,
where he got his master's, and so I stopped taking the amphetamines and immediately started to gain weight. [*Here
Laura is blaming her weight problem on the lack of amphetamines.*] It grew slowly, but nevertheless I started to gain.
We got married in August, and I got pregnant the following
January, and I would say from that time I just kept gaining
weight steadily and went from a low of 123 pounds to a high
of 188 pounds. [*Pregnancy is also blamed for the weight
gain.*]

"Since we've been married, I've been on diet after diet,
and never have been able to help myself to get down to any
kind of a goal. [*Failure, again.*] My husband is in the Coast
Guard, so he has in the past been out to sea for long periods
of time. During one of these periods, maybe four years after
we were married, a little bit more, say six years, I went to
Weight Watchers and took off maybe sixteen to twenty
pounds, and I felt and looked good. As soon as my husband
came back, I just went right back into the same old habits
and very quickly put on all the weight and maybe a little bit
more that I had lost. [*Is Laura's husband a barrier?*]

"The second successful diet that I went on was after I got
professional help from a psychiatrist. At that time we were
living in Bowie, Maryland, and I had difficulty relating to
this psychiatrist on a one-to-one basis, and we weren't really
getting anyplace, and she suggested that I go into group
therapy, and I did that, and that really seemed to be very
helpful. I can't explain why it was helpful. I always felt that
all the other people there had problems that were far greater
than mine, and they probably thought the same thing about
me. But anyway, it was interesting, and I enjoyed it, and
somehow I started going on a diet, and I lost about forty-two
pounds on that particular diet, and I looked good, and I felt

extremely well. I was very happy with myself. [*Laura doesn't have to be fat; she can lose weight.*]

"About this time I had a part-time job working for three internists, and although I was very busy between that job and my home, I really did enjoy working. At this point, I hurt my back while at work, and the outcome was that I stayed home for six weeks and just about stopped dieting and started to slowly put on weight again. [*The back injury becomes a barrier.*] And I was never really able to get back to the diet, and left Bowie, Maryland, and came here to Hawaii. We've been here a little over two years, and I've tried two or three different diets since we've been here and successfully lost eighteen pounds one time, and very quickly put that back on also. Throughout all of our married life my husband has been very supportive of me and of my problems, and I've been able to talk about them and I think I've come to the stage of my life where I'm feeling much more certain that I can overcome my problems, and I feel that I owe a great deal to him because he has been so very supportive and understanding. It's almost like talking to a psychiatrist when I talk to him because we are able to communicate in this way very easily. [*These are all assets.*]

"Just a little over a week ago, my husband and I went to a marriage encounter with a group for a weekend, and this was a big lift to me. It gave me a wonderful feeling of self-confidence, a happy feeling in my marriage. Able to relate to my husband, and he to me even better than we were able to do before this encounter weekei 1 and more, it gave me a reason for living and just a joy in being alive that I haven't had before. Just made me feel that I really loved my husband, my children, my family, and just was happy to be alive. This experience has given me a lot of comfort and a lot of strength, and I feel very confident that it is going to be a positive force in helping me to lose weight. [*Even more assets for Laura.*]

"I think I could profit by learning a new behavior to get

over this feeling of being a loser, and I feel that this, to me, is synonymous with losing weight. If I can lose weight, it will be because I've learned to have better feelings about myself. I want to reach a goal of 120 pounds. [*A stated goal.*] In the past, I've set goals for myself and there have been any number of reasons that I could name for failing to meet them, like I would suddenly gain weight around the time of my period and become discouraged, or I tend to put on weight easily just by eating something a little bit salty and that would discourage me, or I would be really very good about dieting and still not lose weight and that would discourage me. So somewhere along the way, I would feel discouraged. Maybe I would be overtired and that would lessen my ability to stick with the diet. At any rate, I would start nibbling a little here and there, and before I knew it I was off the diet completely again. [*Past failures.*]

"My goal is to be able to learn a way that will get me over these kinds of feelings—unhappy with myself and with the diet, and the feelings of discouragement. I want to learn a way to reach my goal, and I really want to look attractive and feel good. Above all, I want to have a good self-image.

"In replaying this tape, I realized that I did not touch on one portion of my life that may or may not be a significant factor. [*Laura was listening to herself.*] I strongly feel that it is time to stop living in the past and worrying about what my relationship was to my mother or to my father. Whatever that relationship was, I should now be able to get over that, over the feelings that those relationships led to, and I hope that I can learn to forget the negative feelings that some of these relationships created in me. [*When the past doesn't work, leave it alone. It can't be changed.*]

"My mother was a strong and determined person. And still is. And it was largely due to her determination that we arrived in this country. My mother was and is a very beautiful woman, five feet six, which makes her about four inches taller than I am. In her younger years, she was offered a number of modeling jobs. She has always been very concerned about her appearance. She has never been heavy. She is a very chic and smart dresser. Even in rough times, she would prefer to have one expensive dress, expensive and chic, rather than several cheap dresses. I always looked up to my mother and felt very proud of her. I don't feel that my mother was able to show her love outwardly, if indeed she was able to feel much love for her children. I think that she did and still does feel much closer to my sister than to me. I can't tell you exactly why that is, except that my sister was able to accomplish more in her younger years. In high school she was the salutatorian of her class and she was very popular and was maybe the kind of things that my mother would have liked from me and was disappointed I wasn't able to produce.

"I was just twenty-one years old when my father passed away, and I feel that I never got very close to him. He was terribly busy because during the war years he was the only doctor in the little town where we lived in upstate New York, and he was so very busy that he never had much time for his children, although I feel that he was able to show more outward love to both of his daughters than my mother was able to show. I did get quite close to my sister, because she was living in New York City. She was married when I went to nursing school, and so we had a pretty good relationship, and she had two children, and I was around when they were born. I felt useful. I could help take care of the children, and I feel that we had a good relationship. I feel closer to my sister than I do to my mother.

"I feel very close to my husband, and I think we have a very good relationship. [*Another asset.*] In the past I felt that I lacked the physical demonstration of love from him, which he does have trouble in showing. Little things like holding hands, giving me a kiss or a smack on the behind. That kind of physical demonstration. But particularly since our marriage encounter weekend, that has markedly improved and really makes me feel very good and gives me very warm feelings toward him. My relationship to my two daughters, I feel, is very good. I think that I am able to demonstrate my love for them, and they for me. We are able to discuss and to talk, and we have shared some very good times together, and I enjoy being a mother, although there are times when it would be nice not to be straddled with all the responsibilities that go along with it.

"My husband and I took a course, a TA [*transactional analysis*] course, last year through the University of Hawaii, and I think that has helped the communications in the whole family. It makes me realize where I'm coming from at times. I tend to lose patience easily, and I can look at myself now and realize where I'm coming from and review the situation in my mind and come up with a more adult-like solution. [*Another asset.*] I don't think this works constructively for me all the time, but it has been a great deal of help, and is another reason that I think I'm right at this point to learn a new way of life that will ultimately bring me to the role that I'm seeking."

As I mentioned earlier, Laura is almost a textbook example. As a youngster, she learned that eating "everything" earned approval. During the times when she did lose weight, she did so without learning a new eating behavior. She used pills. When she stopped taking pills, she gained back the weight, thus developing a sense of failure. Then, too, she continued to have a poor self-image. Along with this, she was clinging to the past, worrying about it.

Once Laura recognized her problem and set a goal, she was on her way. *By making and listening to the tape,* Laura discovered she had many assets; she was an able, competent woman. By focusing on her assets and her talents, she developed excitement and enthusiasm for her life. She became excited about learning new eating behavior and losing weight.

25

This Could Be You: An Interview with an Eating Winner

Earlier in the book I described a young woman, Marcia, who called me late one afternoon because she was about to eat a pie in reality even though she did not want it. I suggested she eat the pie in her head, and she described the process in great detail. So much detail, in fact, that I lost interest in an ice cream sundae. There is more to Marcia than just a good imagination—she is a real eating winner. That is why I want to tell you more about her.

When twenty-four-year-old Marcia first called for an appointment, she said she wanted to have her jaw wired shut so she could not eat. The first time Ron Pion and I saw Marcia she weighed 248 pounds. "Desperate" is the only way to describe her. She had all but checked out of living. To avoid people, she worked nights for a baby-sitting service. To hide her shame over her eating, she made sure all the blinds were drawn in her apartment before raiding the refrigerator. She hated the way she looked but was convinced she would "never never" lose weight by herself. In spite of all the reducing schemes she followed, she did not accomplish her goal to lose weight. And Marcia had tried everything—including a couple of programs that Ron and I had never heard of.

We do not wire jaws, and we do not refer people to other doctors who use this procedure. When Marcia walked in the door, Ron and I greeted her with a series of incoherent sounds. Marcia just stood there giggling and asked, "Are you two crazy?" We assured her we were not, but that we were only demonstrating life with a wired jaw.

"I see your point," she said. "Okay, it's not for me—but what is?" At this point, she looked as if she were going to cry, but she did seem interested when we explained our methods. "I have nothing to lose" was her attitude.

Marcia actually had a great deal to lose—125 pounds. As I write this, she's lost 78 pounds. From the very first day, Marcia approached her weight loss program with enthusiasm, and has had nothing but success.

Ron Pion made a series of video tapes with Marcia, and I am including extracts from her first and second taping sessions because she is such an inspiration and model to others. Today, Marcia is a changed woman—she lives life fully and is now working during the day as a nursery school teacher. More important, Marcia is a happy, proud young woman with a history of successful weight loss. Marcia's story could very well be yours!

The first taped interview between Ron Pion and Marcia was made about three weeks after she started on a weight loss program. She decided to stay on course because she found that learning new eating behavior was not as difficult as she thought it would be.

RON: I get the idea you learned to be the way you are, and that you don't like being that way. Tell me what it is you dislike about your weight.

MARCIA: I'm fat and sloppy-looking. I can't improve my looks with makeup, clothes, or anything. I just don't look good.

R: Is this your first attempt at losing weight?

M: Oh, no. It seems like I've been on dozens of programs.

R: Did any of them work?

M: I'd lose a few pounds here and there, but then I'd go off and gain back more than I lost.

R: What was the last program you were on?

M: It was a thing with shots. Something to do with a serum. I had these shots and was given a diet to follow—a chicken would starve on it. But I followed it for about three weeks and lost maybe twenty pounds.

R: Why did you stop?

M: I got so sick, and then I started to break out in a rash. I had this awful rash on my arms, my legs, and my face; but I wanted to stick this thing out because I paid $243 for the shots. But I was so sick that I had to stop.

R: How much money have you spent on reducing schemes?

M: I guess between $300 and $500. Pills, shots, you name it, I've tried it.

R: Some people feel seeing a doctor isn't as helpful as joining a group. How do you feel about groups?

M: I was uncomfortable with the group. I felt that I didn't belong there, even though they talked a lot of sense. But I didn't feel I belonged there.

R: Why do you think you're fat?

M: I'm fat because I eat too much.

R: Why do you eat too much?

M: When I'm bored, I eat. When I'm disgusted or mad at myself, I eat. Food is always my pick-me-up. I like to eat. I fall back on food. Especially sweets. I love sweets.

R: What is your favorite food?

M: Pie. When I know pie is there, I want to eat it.

R: What kind of pie?

M: Chocolate cream pie. But now at least I've started to tell myself that the pie won't taste as good as I think it will, and I won't enjoy eating it. I'm beginning to believe that—really believe.

R: Do you dream about food?

M: Oh, yes. All the time. When I get a craving like for a pizza, something I don't normally eat, I get these weird cravings, then I try to sleep; and I dream about the food I want. Then I wake up, and I go and eat it.

R: Are you doing anything to stop these cravings?

M: I try drinking a glass of water.

R: Does it work for you?

M: Oh, yes. If I drink a glass of water, the craving goes away.

R: When you do eat now, are you doing anything different?

M: I look in a mirror now when I eat so I can see myself.

R: How do you feel when you watch yourself eat?

M: Scared—it's awful to see me eating. I never realized how ugly my eating behavior is. I don't want to look like that.

R: Are you using any other new behaviors?

M: Well, one thing I'm doing now—if I feel I have to have some food, I get it and chew it, but I don't swallow it. I just chew it and spit it out.

R: Does this work?

M: Yes, it works for me. Just chewing the food takes the craving away—I can taste it, but I don't have to swallow it. I have also learned to chew a lot longer and more slowly. Sometimes I get tired of chewing, but I never really chewed before. I learned I don't have to swallow everything I put in my mouth. I learned to like, and I mean really like, vegetables. Oh, yes, and now I put my knife and fork down between bites. I never did that before, either. That fork was always going. I think the secret is convincing yourself you like these things. I just told myself I like carrots, and in a few days I did like them. You have to keep telling yourself, "I like carrots—carrots taste good."

R: How much do you want to weigh?

M: 125 pounds.

R: Describe yourself as you are now.

M: Fat, lumpy legs, big hips, a waistline like a man's, big shoulders, and a fat face.

R: Can you picture how you would look at 125 pounds?

M: Oh, yes, there's a picture in my mind right now. It wasn't there when I first saw you, though. I just saw me as fat.

R: Tell me how you see yourself looking at 125 pounds.

M: I see slender legs, small hips, small waistline, small arms and shoulders, and a cute face. I like me very much.

R: You've lost a few pounds already, haven't you?

M: Yes, four or five.

R: Has it been easy?

M: A lot easier than I thought it would be. Much easier than the other things I tried. I think it's because I'm doing different things now. I'm eating vegetables now, and before I wouldn't touch them. I found out I liked carrots, celery, things like that. They're good, and I didn't know they were so tasty. I even like shopping for them.

R: You mentioned you ate when you were bored. What do you do now when you get bored?

M: First, I look for something interesting to do.

R: Does it take long to learn new things?

M: It takes as long as you want it to take. I wanted to get moving, so I learned fast. If you're not interested, it will take a while. I set my own standards. I really want to do these things, so I learned fast because I wanted to.

R: What's wrong with being fat?

M: A lot of things. I feel lazy, always tired, sloppy, shy. I miss out on a lot of things. I like to swim, but I wouldn't be caught dead in a bathing suit. I'd feel embarrassed, self-conscious.

R: How long do you think it will take you to reach 125?

M: Six months to a year.

R: What happens if at the end of that time you weigh only, say, 219?

M: Nothing. I'll keep striving for 125. It will come in time. How long it takes doesn't really matter—just so it comes.

About four months later, Marcia came back for a second interview with Ron. She had lost forty pounds and was thrilled. She was also a young woman who had discovered the joy of living!

R: How much do you weigh now?

M: Today I weigh 210. Since I saw you for the first interview I lost 40 pounds!

R: Terrific! What behavioral assets did you acquire that allowed you to lose 40 pounds in about four months?

M: Learning how to eat good foods like vegetables. Learning to eat slowly and really chew. Today when I want to eat, instead of rushing to the refrigerator, I drink a couple of glasses of water—not fast, either. I sort of sip them slowly. And I don't say I'm on a diet or anything like that. I just say I'm losing weight.

R: What did you do, like yesterday, that let you lose weight in contrast to, say, last March?

M: I picked foods that would allow me to lose weight. I picked cucumbers for lunch and really enjoyed them. And I mean I liked them!

R: How much food are you eating at one time?

M: Very little. I find the longer I chew, the less food I need. Today I can go from breakfast till lunch without a snack. Before, I would have one or two between-meal snacks, but now I'm just not hungry, and when I'm not hungry, I don't eat.

R: How do you feel about cravings now?

M: It's not such a big thing with me any more. They're not assets with me so I leave them alone. I want assets, not liabilities.

R: Do you still have liabilities?

M: Yes, I guess these cravings are liabilities.

R: What do you do about them?

M: I sit down and fantasize I'm eating the food, or I think about something else, anything else.

R: What works better—thinking about something else or fantasizing?

M: Fantasizing works better because thinking is a type of doing behavior just like physical eating is, only on a different level, or at least it is to me.

R: Anything else get in your way?

M: I guess people do. I feel I need some back-up. At home I'm getting a negative attitude about losing. I'm ignoring it.

R: What do you want to learn that will assist you even more toward your goal?

M: I'd like to learn more about exercise. And how to learn to cope with other people. How to be even more relaxed about life—not take it so seriously.

R: How did you feel about yourself when we looked at the first video tape?

M: Disgusted. I didn't realize how ugly I was with all that fat. I didn't like that me at all! Now at 210 it's not great, but it's better than it was, and I know it's going to be even better.

R: Was that the real you on the first tape?

M: No, not today, it isn't.

R: What do you like about this weight?

M: For the first time I went to a store, a regular store, not a place for fat people, and bought a suit. They had it right there on a rack. I could never do that before. It's so nice not to have to wear those sacks for fat people like I wore the first day I came in here.

R: How do you feel about your 40-pound loss?

M: I feel wonderful! I feel I've really accomplished something. I'm a new person because I know I'm going all the way. It's such a thrill having come this far, and I don't think I could ever turn back. I know I can do it. I've proved it to myself.

R: Have you slipped at all?

M: A couple of times.

R: How did you feel?

M: Very guilty. I didn't like the way I felt. So now I know if I slip I'm going to feel guilty. Rather than have a negative feeling, I don't slip. That's all there is to it.

R: Do you tell yourself how wonderful you are?

M: Oh, yes! Every day. And I don't feel silly about it, either. When I first started it, I felt dumb, but now I really believe I am a terrific person. It's a fact with me, and there's nothing dumb about facts. I'm just telling myself the truth.

R: Do you like doing this?

M: Very much, because I don't have to wait for other people to compliment me. I do it myself. I don't have to depend on other people for compliments.

R: Do you weigh yourself a lot?

M: Every day. The first thing in the morning and the last thing at night.

R: Do you ever want to look the way you did last June?

M: No, never again! That's not the real me, and I don't want it.

R: I noticed you changed your hair style. Is there a reason?

M: Yes, because now I dress differently, and I wanted a hair style to match. I feel good about the way I can dress now. I bought a skirt the other day, and I never wore a skirt in my life!

R: Is it exciting?

M: Very much so!

R: Has anything else changed?

M: I'm smoking less now. I'm working days now and I have more on my mind, so I have less time to eat and less time to smoke. I feel so much in control of myself.

R: Do you have anything to share with other people about weight?

M: Yes, I do, because I used to think that I couldn't do it by myself. I would have to go into a hospital, or somebody would have to hold my hand. But that's not so. You have to do it by yourself. If somebody does it for you, it doesn't mean as much. The best feeling comes when you do it by yourself. And that's what I did. I just decided I was going to slim down, and I'm doing it.

R: If somebody asked you, "How can others lose weight?" what would you answer?

M: By learning. First of all, you have to stop learning what you've been learning. It means learning new methods, and stop using the old ones.

R: How is your self-esteem at this point?

M: Very, very high. Before I lost weight, I thought of myself as a fat slob, but today I know I'm a good person. I've proved it. I've lost 40 pounds, and I'm going to lose more.

And she did, too. As I write this, Marcia weighs 170 pounds! And she still intends to weigh 125.

26

From One Success to Another

Back in the days when I was fat, buying clothes was a drag.
I avoided it whenever possible. As I've said, I like clothes.
But I could never find anything that I liked that fit. And
when I did find something that I admired, it didn't come in
my size. The men's clothing industry, like the women's, does
not pay much attention to the overweight. So when I did go
shopping, my choice was limited. There were only one or
two styles in one or two colors. If I didn't like what was
shown to me, that was tough. And after a while what I bought
had to be let out anyway. There was even a time when I had
to have suits custom-made. Everything in the shops was too
tight—that's how heavy I was.

Of course I rationalized this problem. For one thing, I did
not need many clothes. Honolulu is an informal city. Besides
that, I was a doctor and during the hours I was at the hospital
I wore scrub suits. Who knew or cared what was under the
scrub suit? Not that I didn't admire the latest European designs. I did. And when I could find a designer suit that fit, I
was like a kid with a new toy. But this did not happen very
often, and after I lost weight my wardrobe was skimpy.

I had a lot of my everyday things—slacks, clothes like that
—taken in. But I was still nervous about updating my ward-

robe. Not because I doubted I would stay thin. Oh, no, I knew I was not going to be fat again. I was embarrassed. I did not know a thing about color coordination, what shirt looked best with what suit. You see, there is really no such thing as having no problems. Solve one problem and another presents itself. When I was heavy, my problem was finding clothes that fit. Now that I was thin, my problem was coordinating an outfit so I looked well in what I was wearing. I had no idea where to begin, so I kept putting off a shopping trip. A gynecological conference in Boston, where I was participating as a faculty member of a seminar, took care of that.

Boston is not the most informal of cities, and medicine is not the most informal of professions. But I did not have much in my closet to choose from. I packed a few pairs of slacks, some shirts, and a pair of sandals and flew off to Boston. One evening there was a dinner at the Harvard Club, and there I was without the proper clothes. I spent a frantic hour trying to borrow things. The blue suit was too short, and the brown shoes were too small. A few hours in those shoes and I thought I would never walk again. The only spare shirt had French cuffs, but nobody had an extra pair of links. The tie was the ugliest thing I had ever seen and a bit too narrow for my taste. I don't know how I looked to others, but as I looked in the mirror something told me I would not make the list of the Ten Best Dressed Men.

The next morning I was back in my slacks and sandals. At least these clothes fit. During a coffee break I walked past one of the tables and noticed a list of faculty names. One of the doctors had been making notes next to each name. Ordinarily I would not have paid attention, but I saw a comment next to my name. This particular doctor had written next to Reich, Laurence, "sandals?" Oh, yes, question mark and all. I want to stand out in a crowd but not because I am wearing sandals. It was time to buy new clothes—I could not avoid it any longer.

I was a successful loser. Now I wanted to be a successful dresser. I made a few inquiries among people whose taste in clothes I admired. What I was doing was picking another model, this time for my wardrobe instead of my weight. Wilkes-Bashford of San Francisco was recommended as one of the best men's clothing stores in the country. This was very convenient, because I try to get to San Francisco as often as possible. Two of my closest friends, Stu and Davita, live there. Their daughter Raina is my godchild, and I try to see them several times a year. While updating my wardrobe, I could spend time with people who mean a great deal to me.

Off I went to San Francisco and Wilkes-Bashford. I had one of the best times I have ever had because not only did I discover the pleasure of choosing, but I also found another Trusted Other. At Wilkes-Bashford, I started talking to one on the salesmen and I explained my problem. For so many years I had been unable to dress the way I wanted to that I did not know where to begin. Barry was more than happy to help me out and share with me his experience and knowledge.

Gradually, I achieved another of my goals—a fashionable wardrobe of European designer clothes. Shopping for clothes became as exciting as shopping for food. I acknowledged myself for my achievement, but very shortly I was to acknowledge myself for another achievement. I had done so well that one of the leading names in the men's fashion industry acknowledged me!

During a trip to New York City I had ordered a suit from a leading designer for men, Piero Dimitri. He has won three Coty Awards during his career—richly deserved, because his designs are excellent. The suit I ordered needed minor alterations, and I really did not have much time. I explained the situation, and as a favor I was given a fitting appointment on Labor Day. When I arrived at the fitting room I found a skeleton staff, and Dimitri himself. Even on a holiday, he was in his fitting room tinkering with a new design.

I was measured for the alterations and was about to leave

when Dimitri said to one of his assistants, "I've gone as far as I can without a model. I need a model to try this on!" Casting his eyes around the fitting room in frustration, Dimitri spotted me. Raising his expressive hands, he said, "Ah, you will do perfectly. Would you be kind enough to model these trousers so I can see how they will hang? I am designing a suit for a man with your physique. This suit will be worn by a man of your height and weight."

Only three years before, I had been a mound of flesh. If I had walked into Dimitri's showroom when I was fat, he might have invited me to leave. Dimitri does not want blobs wearing his clothes. Now he was telling me I was an ideal model! A designer who is a perfectionist par excellence was asking me to do him a favor! A man who once said, "I would rather that my clothes were recognized by the workmanship than by the label."

I had gone from one success to another. I was a successful loser, and now I was a successful dresser. Success begets success. This is something I learned when I learned I did not have to be fat. I think it is something you will learn too. A successful weight loss will be only the beginning. Achievement can follow achievement as naturally as day follows night. Before you know it, you can have a large assortment of positive features to admire and acknowledge.

I am only one success among many, and there is always room for more successful people. The positive world is not just for a select few—it is for everyone who cares to join. And everybody is able to join—if they choose. Why not leave the negative world of −10 to 0 and cross the barrier to the positive world of 0 to +10? You can, if you want.

ABOUT THE AUTHOR

Born in Mount Vernon, New York, Dr. Laurence Reich is a gynecologist and former assistant professor at the University of Hawaii School of Medicine. He was the first Ortho Fellow in Family Planning and Sexuality and has done medical research in Africa. Dr. Reich is most interested in enhancing opportunities for learning about health and the attainment of personal satisfaction as well as the process of problem solving and the promotion of well-being. He has successfully applied the methods described in this book in his work with overweight individuals and groups. He maintains his home (and his trim weight) in Honolulu.

ENERGISTICS $1.75
BUSTER CRABBE

Simple shape-up exercises that achieve visible results in the shortest possible time without special equipment. The man who knows what fitness means charts the path to better health, more energy, youthful appearance, even longer life, without self-denial, discomfort or boredom.

THE INSTANT SLEEP METHOD $1.95
L. AQUINO, M.D.

Learn the safe way to sleep soundly and wake up refreshed. An expert will help you analyze your personal sleeping problems, solve them by changing old habits, and learn proper procedures for relaxed sleep with a medically proven program.

HOW TO GET THE MOST FOR
YOUR MEDICAL DOLLAR $1.95
JORDAN C. LEWIS

This guide to saving money on your health, medical and dental bills tells you how to select a physician, save money in hospitals and on medication, judge a competent dentist, buy the right kind of health insurance, choose a nursing home, take advantage of clinics and other health services, and much more.

EST: THE MOVEMENT AND THE MAN $1.95
PAT R. MARKS

Have you tried everything from psychotherapy to encounter groups to TM, with no results? Are you unhappy and frustrated with life and do you want to change it? Learn how *est* (Erhard Seminars Training) works and how it can help you, and learn about Werner Erhard, the man who created, organized and runs *est*.

20 MINUTES A DAY TO A MORE
POWERFUL INTELLIGENCE $1.95
ARBIE M. DALE, PH.D.,
with LEIDA SNOW
A step-by-step program for improving reading skills, training memory, enlarging vocabulary, developing creative powers, solving problems faster and heightening perceptions.

MASTERS AND JOHNSON EXPLAINED $1.95
NAT LEHRMAN
The most comprehensive and complete report available of the theories and techniques developed during two decades of sex research. Written in clear, nontechnical language, it will be of aid to millions who have yet to realize their full sexual potential.

SEX FOREVER:
The Key to Male Sexual Longevity $1.95
RAPHAEL CILENTO, M.D., with NEIL FELSHMAN
A scientifically valid, nontechnical guide to sexual fulfillment for the rest of your life. A few simple steps will not only double your sexual pleasure now but will also practically guarantee the kind of long-term sex life you dream about.

THE SANTINI REPORT
ON WOMEN'S SEXUALITY $1.95
ROSEMARIE SANTINI
Researched from 1000 face-to-face interviews, women finally tell what they really want from sex—and how they get it. This human and highly informative book gives a new and greater dimension to female eroticism.